Reiki's Highest Potential

Exploring Original Usui Reiki to
Become Your Highest Potential
Including Eastern & Western
Philosophies
Manuals 1, 2 &

Reiki's Highest Potential

Exploring Original Usui Reiki to
Become Your Highest Potential
Including Eastern & Western
Philosophies
Manuals 1, 2 & 3

Sarina Korotane

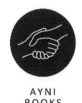

AYNI
BOOKS

Winchester, UK
Washington, USA

JOHN HUNT PUBLISHING

First published by Ayni Books, 2022
Ayni Books is an imprint of John Hunt Publishing Ltd., No. 3 East Street, Alresford
Hampshire SO24 9EE, UK
office@jhpbooks.com
www.johnhuntpublishing.com
www.ayni-books.com

For distributor details and how to order please visit the 'Ordering' section on our website.

ISBN: 978 1 78904 844 5
978 1 78904 845 2 (ebook)
Library of Congress Control Number: 2020951020

A CIP catalogue record for this book is available from the British Library.

Design: Stuart Davies

UK: Printed and bound by CPI Group (UK) Ltd, Croydon, CR0 4YY
Printed in North America by CPI GPS partners

We operate a distinctive and ethical publishing philosophy in
all areas of our business, from our global network of authors to
production and worldwide distribution.

Contents

This book is dedicated to my love, Harvey. Thank you for all your support, for designing and illustrating the symbols for this book, but most of all, for giving me the time and space to write and finish this book.

I would also like to thank all of you who read this book. Take what you will and adapt it to suit *you*, for your unique highest good, to reach your own unique highest potential. Do not be afraid of where Reiki will lead you. Sometimes the journey feels dark as we explore and try to heal our deepest traumas, but it is also a wonderful and enlightening journey. I wish you well on your healing journey, on all the journeys you will take as a healer, and I thank you for sharing a part of mine.

Inscription on Mikao Usui's headstone:

If Reiki can be spread throughout the world it will touch the human heart and the morals of society. It will be helpful for many people, not only healing disease, but the Earth as a whole.

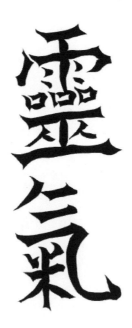

'Reiki' in Japanese

Introduction

When we are truly ready, the universe will always bring us opportunities to grow, to evolve, and to become our individual highest potential. Then, when everything seems to be flowing just as we want, life again challenges us with more to learn. Finding our highest potential is an ongoing journey and part and parcel of being alive, and for me, Reiki is my guide.

Reiki – it's a funny one to explain to people who have no knowledge of energy healing, of which there are many different paths, Reiki being just one. Energy healing is something that many of us give and receive on a daily basis without realising it. It's in the small things, such as a parent's kiss, a friend's embrace, sitting alone in nature feeling at one with the trees, or watching the distant waves of the sea with your love. We are all giving and receiving energy continuously, but most of us just cannot see it with our human eyes. We can, however, feel it. We, as human beings, are able to connect with all the universal energy vibrations around us and utilise them to achieve great things. Reiki can feel like magic, but in truth it's a science which hasn't been explored enough.

Reiki healing is basically a tool (practice/method) used to cleanse energy blocks which cause dis-ease and imbalance within the physical, mental, emotional and energy/spiritual bodies. It's a tool which heals what we don't know needs healing, our deepest traumas and dis-ease. It's a tool which rebalances our energy, aiding the healing of physical issues, grounding us mentally and emotionally, and giving us an energetic/spiritual freedom.

Having been taught Original Usui Reiki, both Eastern and Western philosophies, this is the Reiki I share with you. The book has been structured into the three Reiki Degree manuals and are as I give them to my students. The manuals themselves are guides and structured to give you the basic information for that particular Reiki Degree, including all the meditations and exercises I was taught and still use. They contain both the Western and Eastern philosophies and practical uses for that level of Reiki. I've also included my experiences – how each Reiki Degree took me on a journey and guided me to discover who I was and how to reach my highest potential at a particular moment in my life. This book is a guide on how to use Reiki to heal yourself so you may reach your highest potential – be it your mental and/or emotional life to improve your career or personal relationships, or physical issues, or your personal energy/spiritual life to gain more perspective on who you are on a deeper level.

Reiki is unique to each of us, and each of us will require cleansing and healing at different points in our lives. This book is written for all those interested in Reiki, from Reiki Masters to newcomers, to people who have been attuned but have not practised in a long time. However, if you are new to Reiki, be aware that the information itself does not make you a Reiki Healer; for this you must be 'attuned' and/or 'empowered' by an actual Reiki Master.

There are many people who will find ways to attune themselves and start practising Reiki alone with no Reiki Master to guide them. To these people I would advise that to practise Reiki professionally you do need to be Okuden 2nd Degree trained and have proof of your certificates and lineage. I believe that without some form of guidance from a Reiki Master, many will miss out on the experience and knowledge that a Reiki Master can offer. I do personally recommend getting attuned and/or empowered by a Reiki Master, but I also strongly believe that everyone's Reiki journey is their own. You have to follow your own unique path.

This book does contain the Kotodama and symbols with explanations on how to use them. The Kotodama and symbols are tools which are taught in the 2nd Degree and Master Degree to connect to different Reiki energy frequencies which heal on deeper levels of the physical, emotional, mental and spiritual bodies. Many Reiki Masters may feel that I'm disrespecting the teachings of Original Usui Reiki because I have included them in this book. We are taught that the symbols and Kotodama should be kept secret and sacred. I totally agree with the sacred. The symbols and Kotodama should always be sacred to you and be given the utmost respect when using them.

However, like most symbols that are sacred, you can find everything on the internet if you just look, so I feel it is important in this age that we are open and inviting with our practices because we are in a position to guide others towards healing themselves in a respectful, honest and safe manner. Reiki healing practices have evolved through time, spread throughout the world, developed and become more inclusive, and I feel this needs to continue now more than ever.

Now this may come across as a little dramatic, but I truly believe that we are at a point in our human history where we really need to decide how important the future of this planet is. How important our children's futures are. I truly believe that the world needs more healers, and we can all do our bit to commit to a healthier future for ourselves and, in turn, for others.

With the world looking at unstable political governing and economic crises, division, current and potential wars, environmental damage which might be beyond repair, and pandemics which spread globally at an alarming rate, this is a time when Mother Earth and all her inhabitants need healing, positive energy and balance. I feel that each and every one of us healers makes a little difference each time we send out healing and positive thoughts. Every tiny act of healing, of love, of kindness spreads a little more positive energy into the world and it does make a difference, to someone at least.

To see pain and suffering all we have to do is look at our families, friends, communities, the daily news and, most importantly, in the mirror. If we let our guard down and truly explore all the energy vibrations around and within us, we can sense the blockages and how much cleansing and healing is needed. But before we go out to heal the world, as every Reiki Healer knows, the first and best place to start is with the self. The more we cleanse, rebalance and heal ourselves, the better we are placed to support others to heal, and in turn they are better placed to support others' healing – enabling us individually and together to deal with conflict, drama, and trauma within ourselves, our families and communities.

I was first attuned to Reiki over ten years ago, but my history with energy healing started as a child. I didn't know what it was, just that it was normal to me. As I got older and my life became complicated – as it does with every teenager – I put this down to hormones, and I can with hand on heart say I rebelled against everything and anything that would benefit me and I was attracted to the drama of destruction, as a somewhat normal-ish teenager is.

At some point in my twenties I was drawn to reconnect to energy healing again, but I didn't want to follow any particular path. I just really wanted to explore all the energy healing paths that were open to me and I put my faith in the universe to guide me, but for some strange reason I didn't want to learn Reiki and I avoided it. I think I had a somewhat dubious view of it for no reason at all.

It was at a point in my life in my mid-thirties (I was having a mid-thirties crisis) that the opportunity came to take the Shoden 1st Degree with my Reiki Master, Tiffany Crosara, and I jumped on it, and I have never looked back. Reiki came to me when I was finally ready, and I felt lucky to meet Tiffany because I trusted and felt safe with her. That might seem like a strange thing to say, but at that period in my life I didn't feel safe very often. I did all my Reiki Degrees with her, and one of the main things she taught me was that Reiki itself is your teacher and Reiki will guide you on this lifelong path for your own unique highest good – to reach your own unique highest potential.

Reiki healing has since had a profound effect on my life and has lifted and grounded me when required. In truth, on many occasions I have felt naked and raw, and was forced to truly see my flaws. I was put in situations where I had to learn to really look at my intentions and see the thought patterns and behaviours which I kept returning to, work out what triggered them and focus on healing that part of me. I had to learn to trust myself and push myself to be the person I wanted to be. It's an ongoing journey because that is life. Reiki with all its lessons and healing has allowed me to evolve as a person, as a soul, and I know I will continue to grow and evolve.

I'm now in my late forties and in a wonderful place where I'm aware of just how delicate life is and how all its treasures can so easily be gone. I'm aware that I still have much to learn but also accept this is OK, because I'm also in a place of great experience and connection. I seem to have let go of things: behaviour patterns, people and situations that were once so ingrained in my being, and though I look upon my past with love (sometimes cringing), I no longer desire anything or anyone that brings drama into my life.

Many may think this could just be an age thing, but I've discovered that it's more. With Reiki, I've allowed myself to heal so I can take care of what is really important to me – my mental health, my physical health, my emotional health and my spiritual health. Age and life experience give you much, but healing gives you more. It gives you a very real sense of self, of peace, and a love for living, a passion for life.

I am grateful for what I have, knowing that I have no control over external forces or even sometimes what is happening within my own thoughts or physical body. I'm premenopausal, and although that makes life very interesting and the changes can be uncomfortable, I find I no longer fear these changes, but welcome them because I've earned them. I made it to my late forties! I am entering a new stage in my life and I'm excited that my best years are yet to come.

Healing is a lifelong journey and writing this book is a part of my Reiki journey. The universe (life itself, fate, soul path or maybe just my inner needs) is putting me in a place where I feel vulnerable, where I'm unsure of how to proceed or how it will be received. I'm a procrastinator (which is something I must explore so I can heal this part of me, but yes, I've kept putting it off) and honestly it's been hard at times to just get on with things and finish this book. So I'm trying to see it as going on an adventure and it's a little bit scary and a little bit exciting, but I trust in this journey though I have no idea where it will lead. I know that whenever I need guidance or healing of any kind, or maybe a kick up the bum, I have the ability to cocoon myself in a Reiki bubble and find my peace and the strength to pick myself up and carry on.

Chapter 1

Shoden 1st Degree of Original Usui Reiki

Eastern and Western Philosophies

Introduction

The Shoden 1st Degree is the start of your Reiki journey and it's very much focused on healing the self and practising Reiki on the self for your own highest good. On this Degree, the Reiki Master will connect you to Reiki via Attunements and/or a Reiju Empowerment, giving you the ability to be a channel for Reiki for the rest of your life.

If you are new to any form of energy healing, then this is the first step in getting to know your energetic self and how you are connected to the universe on an energetic level. Having the Attunements and Reiju Empowerments connecting you directly to Reiki energy unblocks and cleanses your energetic body, which in turn cleanses and rebalances the physical, mental and emotional bodies. Taking the Reiki 1st Degree can have a profound effect on your well-being and bring changes for your highest good.

The 1st Degree of Original Usui Reiki covers the basics of the different philosophies of Western and Eastern Reiki and how to give yourself Reiki treatments to cleanse and heal. Included are meditations and energy exercises and general guidance, including using Reiki with crystals or treating pets, plants, and general spaces such as your home.

These are all tools to explore once you have been given the basics, and most of your learning will come after the Degree. If you continue to practise Reiki, get to know all the energies and how they feel, it will become second nature to use Reiki in every aspect of your life.

Many Reiki students only complete the Shoden 1st Degree and for many that is all they need. Shoden is focused on the 'self', about healing and cleansing you for your own highest good. By taking the Shoden Degree you're investing in yourself, your well-being, your present and future for yourself, and that is a gift which only you can give yourself.

What Is Original Usui Reiki and Reiki Healing?

So what exactly is Reiki? Well, *Rei* is the Japanese word for 'universal' and *ki* is the Japanese word for 'energy'. 'Reiki' is basically the 'universal energy' that vibrates and flows through every living thing that is fundamental to life as we know it, and beyond what we think we currently know. Within this universal energy, Reiki, there are many different frequencies, and once you've been initiated to these, you can connect to them via 'intention' to heal and cleanse. Intention is key to healing.

We also know this energy by other names; for example, in India it is called *Prana*, in China it's called *Chi*, and William Reich called it 'orgon energy'. Scientists today are discovering new and different energies that vibrate all around us, many of which were known to our ancestors. We may not fully understand it, but once initiated to Reiki, you can feel it and how it connects you to all the universal energy frequencies.

Reiki – the universal energy itself – is not aligned with any religion and it is not particularly a spiritual path; however, people of all cultures, religious backgrounds and ages have connected and used this energy for benefit in their own ways. There are texts that discuss how the Hindu god Shiva gifted the universal healing energy to humans so it may be used by all. There are texts which describe how Jesus, on his travels to India and Tibet, was taught how to use the universal energy to heal others. Many cultures throughout time would have passed on this information via word of mouth, and the actual history of energy cultivation is lost in time. Accessing the universal energy to connect for healing and spiritual guidance has been achieved by many via meditation, spiritual rituals, Attunements and Reiju Empowerments, and even strong emotions.

Original Usui Reiki itself is the method and practice that was developed and used by Mikao Usui and has its roots in Japanese culture and Buddhist teachings. He initiated and taught his students how to connect with the universal energy to release personal energy blockages and remove dis-ease. Reiki is for the self, but being a Reiki Healer also enables you to direct healing to another person, animal, plant, location, situation or even a different time period. Energy healing is universal and accessible to everyone, but it should be recognised that Reiki will not cure a terminal illness, and it will not magically get rid of mental illness or physical disabilities. However, it will aid healing and guide you to some peace of mind, and maybe lift some pain and discomfort.

What makes Reiki healing different from other energy healing practices is that a Reiki Master will open a channel between you and the universal energy and connect you directly to Reiki. This was originally given by Usui to recipients as a Reiju Empowerment. A student of Usui developed Attunements, which spread globally and are used in Western Reiki. Once you have been empowered or attuned you are able to connect to the universal energy and practise Reiki healing at will for life.

There are many different paths and practices of energy healing and there is no right or wrong way because it is about the connection you individually feel. Reiki will fit into your life as you need it to, but the more you practise, the stronger the connection and the more Reiki healing you receive.

The Shoden Cleansing
In Western Usui Reiki, Attunements are given by a Reiki Master to initiate a student and connect Reiki directly to the individual's chakra system. The seven major chakras are initiated; however,

all the chakras go through a cleansing which can take up to six months or longer. In Japanese Usui Reiki, Reiju Empowerments are used to initiate and connect Reiki directly to the individual, and the cleansing period is based on personal development which can take a lifetime.

After being initiated and connected to Reiki on each Degree, the Reiki Master and students embark on a 21-day Reiki cleanse, during which a self-treatment is given each day to cleanse personal energy. It's really important to stick with the cleansing for the full 21 days, but it can be difficult to complete because of all the effects of the cleansing. If at any point you need a break, take it and then restart the whole 21 days again.

The cleansing takes place over two periods of time, the first being the 21-day period during the self-treatments which is called the 'inner change'. The second period is called 'the outer change' and this can take up to six months or longer as it works on deeper and often hidden trauma and dis-ease.

The cleansing period is unique for each individual and so each person will experience different forms of cleansing. They could be flu-like symptoms, headaches, spots, rashes, upset stomach, depression, sadness, extreme tiredness, or on the other side, a lightness of step, walking taller, feeling incredibly happy and carefree, having more mental clarity, or nothing at all. Other experiences may include heightened sensitivity, whether it is emotional, psychic or physical such as sensitivity to smells or noise, or rejecting junk food or smoking. It is unique for each individual.

With the Shoden 1st Degree, changes often occur on a physical level. What no longer serves you in a physical way – for example an illness, your immediate physical environments (place of residence or work) or immediate physical relationships – can change by just healing the thoughts and beliefs that can cause dis-ease. People experience shifts for the better in their physical body and outer life, and with Shoden, the cleansing is easier to see than with the Okuden or Master Degrees because the changes are so physical.

I mentioned before that I never really had an interest in learning Reiki and it's true, but then at a point in my mid-thirties when I was changing jobs, moving to a different city and literally just all over the place mentally and emotionally, I came to the conclusion that I did not know who I was any more. I felt at the time that I had made so many bad decisions in my life that I couldn't trust myself and I was utterly lost. I made one last decision and that was to leave all my decisions up to the universe and let the universe guide me. I can admit that at the time, I didn't really care what decisions were made for me; I had no passion for life.

Then a friend called and asked if I wanted to tag along to a tarot reading and I thought, *The universe sent this to me, so why not?* I booked a tarot reading too and the tarot reader told me that I seemed to be stuck in a cycle in which I was remembering the remembering of memories and that they had become warped by my own remembering. Basically, I was spending so much time focusing on feeling insecure and unsafe that I wasn't giving myself a chance to actually look at facts without being emotional. I was, in a way, indulging in playing the victim. I suppose I should have been a little offended by this, but strangely the guidance he gave me felt positive, like a light had been switched on and I was suddenly given permission to stop being down on myself, but focus on trying to be happy again – to feel alive.

As I walked out of the room, I came across a leaflet for the Shoden 1st Degree and again I felt like the universe was making another decision for me, so I booked it there and then and I never looked back. The Shoden 1st Degree blew my mind because it felt so incredible to actually physically feel this connection to the universe. I carried on living in the mindset of 'the universe will make my decisions', and I took whatever opportunity showed up. I was offered a good temp position in London and as that was coming to a close, I received an offer for a job working in the Middle East and the timing was perfect.

Four months after taking my Shoden 1st Degree, I was physically removed from everyone and everything I knew. I found myself living in the Middle East working on a construction site alongside members of the UK Ministry of Defence and it was hard (they have so many rules – and I don't like rules), but the experience and personal growth resulted in major changes to my mindset and thought patterns. The tarot reader had told me that I needed to just let the past be the past and stop holding on to pain and hurt, and then I was dumped with a bunch of soldiers who only lived in the moment. No tomorrow – no yesterday. Just today and this particular moment.

I learned a lot from these soldiers; they taught me how precious my life is and how privileged I am to be alive. It was a group of soldiers who taught me how to accept myself and be at peace with who I am but to always improve on my flaws. I learned from these soldiers how to let go of hurt and pride, and really laugh at myself. They taught me how to look for the beauty in each moment and to live in that moment. They taught me how to acknowledge and honour my past, to embrace my experiences, good and bad, and see them as positives. I realised that their viewpoint came from the knowledge that they could be sent to war at any given moment, and so they made the absolute most of 'now' with an urgency that I now admire.

The strange thing is that they never realised the positive impact they made on my life. They, on a daily basis, made fun of me, teased me, and looked after me. I found that I stopped blaming others for pain that I had been holding on to, because that choice to hold on to that pain – well, that was my choice, and it was time to let go. I learned to look into the mirror and see that I was the one holding myself back from living my life, from being in the now. My Shoden cleansing period, though extremely hard at times, made me understand that my trauma was a part of me and I could learn from it, grow from it, and be a stronger me. I actually began to honour myself and my life and I did not know what that meant before.

I've stated that the normal cleansing period lasts for about six months. I really think my Shoden cleansing lasted much longer, maybe a year and six months, maybe more... Sometimes even now, I feel that I'm still learning from that period all those years ago. The thing about self-healing is that it really is an ongoing journey and not a single blast of enlightenment. It's a long, slow process of healing that spreads from the deepest depths of our souls to reach our hearts, minds and physical well-being, and it's a journey that goes on and on and on.

As those soldiers taught me, living is a privilege, and regardless of how bleak it can seem at times, we all have the power to heal, to grow and to become our highest potential.

The History of Reiki

All forms of Reiki healing originate from Original Usui Reiki; however, what we know generally as Usui Reiki in the West is not what Usui actually taught in Japan. When Reiki was first introduced to the West, the story of Reiki was adapted to suit different cultural trends, lifestyles and perspectives, but most importantly, one of the consequences of World War Two was that anything associated with Japan or Japanese culture at that time was regarded with distrust in America. So Usui's story had been adapted to suit American values at the time.

In Japan, Reiki had been left relatively untouched, whereas in the West, Reiki continued to adapt and evolve and over the decades developed into many different forms of healing practices. The Western version of the history of Reiki and of Usui himself continued to be taught until the 1990s; then knowledge of Original Usui Reiki as Usui himself taught it was discovered and came to the West.

You will discover by reading different books on Reiki, published at different times, that some have the Western version of Reiki history and others have the Japanese version of Reiki history. I think that the Western version had its benefits because it allowed Reiki to evolve, adapt and spread so it could become available to people all around the globe and this wouldn't have happened if Reiki had remained in Japan.

According to the Western version, Usui was portrayed as the principal of a Christian school near Kyoto, where he was challenged by his students to show them how to heal the way Jesus did – with his hands. Unable to do so, he gave up his position as principal and travelled to the USA to study theology at the University of Chicago (there have never been any records found that he attended this university). After years of studying he returned to Japan to continue his quest to find the answer and went to visit his Zen Master, who told him that if he wanted to know the secrets of healing, he should go to Mount Kurama to meditate and fast for 21 days. It was on the twenty-first day that Usui was given the gift of Reiki.

Usui's actual history became known to the West when Frank Arjava Petter and his Japanese wife went to Japan in 1993 to find the Buddhist origins of Reiki. They traced back the various Reiki streams to the roots of the original system of Usui and discovered not only Usui's handwritten texts on healing techniques but also surviving students who still practised Reiki as Usui had taught it.

With the discovery of Usui's surviving students and texts, it was confirmed that Usui Reiki is a system to find one's spiritual path, to heal oneself, and is rooted in Tendai Buddhism (Mystical Buddhism). Usui was a man with a strong spiritual background which included training in martial arts and energy cultivation. Usui's surviving students described Reiki as 'a path to personal perfection', and the focus was the path to enlightenment. Reiki was for the self, and treating others was something you did along the path.

The actual (Japanese) history of Reiki and Usui himself, as told by his students, states that Mikao Usui, a Tendai Buddhist monk, was born on 15 August 1865 in the village of Taniai-mura (now called Miyama-cho) in the Yamagata district, Gifu prefecture, Kyoto, the former capital of Japan. He died aged 60 on 9 March 1926 from a stroke, leaving behind a wife and two children.

Usui was a well-travelled man who studied to understand the secrets of healing, and he was searching for the 'essence of life' when he asked his Zen Master for guidance. His Zen Master replied that if he wanted to know the secret then he must meditate and fast until he died, and this led him to Mount Kurama, a holy mountain in Japan near Kyoto, which is described as 'the spiritual heart of Japan'. This mountain is a place of many temples where spirits called 'Tengu' are said to have disclosed the secrets of martial arts and fighting to the Samurai.

It was during the third week on this quest for death when Usui, according to his memorial stone, experienced the enlightenment that led to the development of Reiki. Just before dawn, Usui saw a bright light coming straight at him with great speed, which then hit him with such force in the centre of his forehead (third eye) that he was knocked unconscious. Around midday when he regained consciousness, he felt refreshed and energised and rushed down the mountain, but tripped and stubbed his toe, causing an injury. He automatically held his foot, and to his surprise the pain vanished and the injury stopped bleeding and healed. He was excited by this and went to see his Zen Master, who confirmed that Usui had indeed achieved enlightenment and advised him to use this healing ability to heal others and lead them into enlightenment through healing.

Usui returned home and tried the healing on his family, and finding that it produced great results, he decided to share this knowledge. He experimented and developed a method that would enable him to pass on this ability to other people so they too could connect to Reiki to heal. This method is now known as Shin-Shin Kai-Zen Usui Reiki Ryo-Ho or 'The Usui Reiki Treatment Method for Improvement of Body and Mind'. He very much believed that Reiki could be accessed by all living beings and heal them so they may live with a pure and sound mind.

Usui then went to Tokyo and established the Usui Reiki Ryoho Gakkai where he set up seminars to teach Reiki and give Reiju Empowerments to students. They were trained to pursue their spiritual development through healing themselves and others. As part of his teaching, Usui taught Kotodama (chanting sounds, a bit like mantras) so his students could access different healing energies and frequencies. Some students found that they were unable to use the Kotodama, so for those students Usui introduced symbols that were a mixture of Sanskrit and Zen Buddhist symbols.

In 1923 when the Great Kanto Earthquake hit Tokyo, Usui rushed to give Reiki treatments to people in the devastated area. When he found that young beggars kept coming back for healing instead of trying to improve their lives, he introduced 'The Five Principles of Reiki' into the healing method. There are 125 'Waka' poems that he taught with Reiki, but the Five Principles he put together to encourage mindfulness.

Usui had approximately 2000 students between 1922 and 1926, when he died. As he believed that the students should spend as much time as they could to get to know Reiki, most never went further than Shoden 1st Degree or Okuden 2nd Degree. However, before he died he had trained around 20 students to Shinpeden and Shihan Master Teacher level.

The Usui Reiki Ryoho Gakkai is still run today and has around 300 to 400 members; however, it is hard to become a member and apparently they do not practise Reiki on anyone outside of the organisation. Information is hard to obtain in regard to their Reiki practices and theories, but it is important to note that Usui's Reiki did survive outside of the Gakkai and was taught and spread by his students.

Usui initiated Dr Hayashi to the Master Degree in the year he died. Dr Hayashi was an ex-captain in the Imperial Japanese Navy, and as a naval doctor with his medical background, he viewed Reiki from a treatment angle. He founded the Reiki Healing Clinic in Tokyo and initiated Mrs Hawayo Takata (a Japanese lady living in Hawaii) to Master level in 1935; she then spread Reiki to the West.

What we do know about the development of Reiki is that due to the closed membership of the Gakkai, the only way Reiki could have survived and become widespread in Japan was by its reintroduction from the West. Though we do know of students of Usui who did survive and did in turn teach others, it was only a small number of Practitioners. It was via the West that Reiki again began to thrive in Japan once it had become so widespread across the globe.

Western Philosophies and Practice of Original Usui Reiki

When I was first taught Original Usui Reiki, there was a sense that the Eastern approach was deeply spiritual and that the Western outlook focused on relaxing, de-stressing, mental and emotional well-being, and physical treatments. However, I've discovered that it really depends on individuals' belief systems. More people in the West are now open to living a more mindful and spiritual lifestyle without it being religious, and in the East attitudes are also changing and people are taking on a more Western viewpoint in their lifestyles. As the world becomes a smaller place and more knowledge is shared, it has resulted in Reiki healing practices constantly evolving and becoming available to more people of different belief systems.

Reiki in the West evolved and there are many different paths. Western Reiki is more open to change, and we in the West are more open to taking something and adapting it to suit our individual needs. In the West, we have Reiki that is associated with angels, alien beings and pagan belief systems, and they all have their own rituals for connecting to the universal energy. However, most Western Reiki paths work on the auric body and chakra system, and some Reiki organisations only place their hands on certain body areas, and their treatments are timed and very structured.

Western Usui Reiki has had new symbols introduced that are not used in Japanese Original Usui Reiki. There is a spiritual aspect in Western Usui Reiki in that it is based on the auric body and chakra system, which is seen as the spiritual body of the whole person. So it is true to say that most Western Reiki is spiritual and does work on the whole, but it doesn't mean that you need to be spiritual or follow spiritual teachings. You just need to connect and feel the universal energy.

The Auric Body

Every living entity on this planet has its own energy field, and it doesn't stop there. All the rocks, rivers, lands and seas, Mother Earth herself, the other planets and our solar system... literally everything is made up of vibrating energy fields. Everything is somehow connected to the universal energy, and we are all, in our core, an energy field carrying around a body that is made of stardust.

Our personal energy field vibrates and expands beyond our physical bodies and can become clogged with negativity, causing an imbalance which can be felt physically, mentally, emotionally or energetically/spiritually. This personal energy field is also known as your aura or auric body, and this system is rooted in the Indian subcontinent. Its teachings originate in Hinduism, and then as further belief systems developed in Asia, its teachings spread to other Eastern belief systems such as Buddhism. The auric body consists of seven energy layers that extend outwards from our physical body, and our auras are in effect the extension of our bodies or 'the coat of consciousness'. The colours and shapes of our auras change according to our moods, feelings and energy levels; for instance, if someone is feeling depleted, this is likely to be reflected in their aura retracting to about 2 or 3 feet. The normal extension should be about 6 feet, which accounts for our personal space.

The Chakra System

The word *chakra* literally translates from Sanskrit as 'wheel'. The chakras are shown as cone-shaped vortices of energy, which spin and vibrate within the energy body. The human body consists of 7 major chakras, 21 minor chakras, 49 minute chakras and numerous minuscule chakras. The seven major chakras radiate out from different points along the spine to the top of the head, forming a vertical axis. Western Usui Reiki focuses on all of the major chakras as well as the two most important minor chakras, which are found within the palms of the hands.

Chakras penetrate right through our auric body from the front to the back and look like funnels on stems, just like wheels as they spin. In a sense they are described as our ethereal plugs to life, enabling us to connect our energy force with our mental, emotional and physical bodies. As chakras spin they can become clogged with negativity throughout our daily lives, and this can result in negative thoughts, words, situations and so on. Over time, if left untended, this in turn can manifest into a physical, emotional, mental or spiritual/energy imbalance or dis-ease.

When using Reiki to heal or unblock our chakras, we can focus the energy to go straight to the chakra which governs that particular issue or dis-ease, or we can connect and open all our chakras for a thorough cleansing.

THE SEVEN CHAKRA SYSTEM

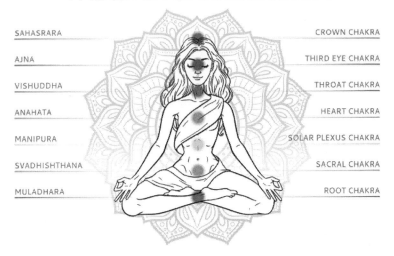

SAHASRARA	CROWN CHAKRA
AJNA	THIRD EYE CHAKRA
VISHUDDHA	THROAT CHAKRA
ANAHATA	HEART CHAKRA
MANIPURA	SOLAR PLEXUS CHAKRA
SVADHISHTHANA	SACRAL CHAKRA
MULADHARA	ROOT CHAKRA

Auric body and chakra system

The seven major chakras are as follows:

The root or base chakra:

- Layer: This is the first layer of the auric body and honours the Earth.
- Colour: Red
- Location: Base of the spine and points down between the legs.
- Function: The root chakra connects with our 'rootedness' or our 'base' survival, which is how to function in the physical world, our will to live and our basic needs.
- Signs of a healthy root chakra: being grounded in life, reliable, steadfast, and having perseverance.
- Signs of an unhealthy root chakra: Mental or emotional imbalance in the root chakra can show itself as aggression or passivity, ruthless ambition or lack of passion, feeling unsupported, insecure or angry.
- Governs: Physically the root chakra governs the hips down,

the coccyx, the adrenals, skin and blood.

The sacral or splenic chakra:

- Layer: This is the second layer of the auric body and honours the Creative.
- Colour: Orange
- Location: Sacrum just under the belly button.
- Function: This chakra connects with sensation and expression such as pleasure, creativity, sexuality and physical enjoyment.
- Signs of a healthy sacral chakra: a cheerful, warm, optimistic, positive demeanour and creative/sexual expression.
- Signs of an unhealthy sacral chakra: Mental and emotional imbalances can occur as blocked creativity, leading to greyness in life, depression, guilt, obsessions and addiction.
- Governs: Physically the sacral chakra governs our reproductive system, intestines, kidneys, urinary tract and lower back.

The solar plexus chakra:

- Layer: This is the third layer of the auric body and honours the Life Force.
- Colour: Yellow
- Location: Just below the rib cage and above the belly button.
- Function: This chakra connects with our will, purpose, confidence, independence and sense of self. It is our centre. Moving from the base chakras into the emotional chakras, this is where people may feel they are having a 'gutful', not being able to 'stomach' something or finding it hard to digest, feeling gutted, or using their gut instinct.
- Signs of a healthy solar plexus: a well-defined sense of self, purpose and clarity.
- Signs of an unhealthy solar plexus: Mental and emotional

imbalances can occur as weakness, dependency, not feeling centred or focused, or self-centredness.

- Governs: Physically the solar plexus governs our digestion, pancreas, muscles, gall bladder and middle back.

The heart chakra:

- Layer: This is the fourth layer of the auric body and honours the Heart.
- Colour: Green and pink
- Location: Centre of the chest.
- Function: This chakra connects with love, compassion, kindness, balance and unity.
- Signs of a healthy heart chakra: an ability to love in a healthy well-balanced manner as well as a healthy self-love.
- Signs of an unhealthy heart chakra: Mental or emotional imbalances occur as mental or emotional abuse of oneself or others, either by conditional or smother love, or an inability to feel or express love, and a lack of heartfelt connection.
- Governs: Physically the heart chakra governs the heart, circulation, upper back, respiratory system, lungs, thymus, arms, hands and immune system.

The throat chakra:

- Layer: This is the fifth layer of the auric body and honours Communication.
- Colour: Blue
- Location: Centre of the throat.
- Function: The throat chakra connects with communication and is the bridge between the emotional and mental/ spiritual states.
- Signs of a healthy throat chakra: clear communication, confidence and being well balanced.

- Signs of an unhealthy throat chakra: Mental or emotional imbalances occur as an inability to speak one's truth, make oneself heard, or loud, dominating or aggressive communication.
- Governs: Physically the throat chakra governs the thyroid, parathyroid, metabolism, ears, nose, throat, mouth and teeth.

The third eye chakra:
- Layer: This is the sixth layer of the auric body and honours the Psychic.
- Colour: Indigo
- Location: Centre of the forehead.
- Function: The third eye chakra connects with our senses, intuition and insight.
- Signs of a healthy third eye chakra: sensitivity, empathy, visionary ability, intuitiveness, psychic and spiritual awareness.
- Signs of an unhealthy third eye chakra: Mental and emotional imbalances occur as confusion, delusion, oversensitivity or lack of sensitivity.
- Governs: Physically the third eye governs the eyes, sinuses, ears, hormones, pituitary gland, brain, face and head.

The crown chakra:
- Layer: This is the seventh layer of the auric body and honours Spiritual Connectedness.
- Colour: Violet or white
- Location: Situated on the top of the head pointing upwards.
- Function: The crown chakra connects with our spirit, our place in the universe and spiritual beliefs.
- Signs of a healthy crown chakra: good connection to the higher self and higher purpose, integrity, mysticism, wisdom, understanding and self-realisation.

- Signs of an unhealthy crown chakra: Mental and emotional imbalances occur as an inability to function well in the physical world, not really being present, being in another world, or a lack of faith or understanding of creation and your place in it, cause and effect.
- Governs: Physically the crown chakra governs the mind, pineal gland, nervous system and the whole body.

How to Feel Your Auric Body

I think it's really important that people are able to feel their own energy vibrations and get to know them. Taking the first step opens your eyes not only to your own energy vibrations but also to all the energy vibrations beyond your own. Practising playing with energy allows you to feel moods on a deeper level, for example another person's or the collective energy of a group of people, or of a location, an animal, and even a situation.

The following exercise enables you to feel your own energy field:

1. Take a seat, either cross-legged on the floor or on a chair with your feet on the floor. Straighten your back as much as you can so your chakras may sit on top of one another in alignment and keep your hands resting upwards on your knees. (If you have difficulties straightening your back with ease, then use cushions to support your back.) Close your eyes if you feel more comfortable doing so.

2. Relax and focus on your breathing. Inhale deeply through your nose and feel the air fill all of your lungs. Exhale from your mouth. Repeat.

3. Now focus on the point just below your navel and visualise your personal energy or just feel for a sensation vibrating within. Feel and focus on the intention to move that energy from your navel up through your abdomen and chest, through your shoulders and down your arms

to the minor chakras in your palms.

4. You should start feeling a sensation in the palms of your hands. This sensation can be heat, or a pins and needles type of feeling, or static electricity. Hold your hands at least 5 inches away from each other, facing each other.

5. Focus and you should be able to feel the air is denser in between your palms. This is your personal energy field. Gently try moving your hands closer to each other and there should be a little resistance.

6. Now play with this energy in between your palms: move them closer together but not touching, then away from each other, and you should be able to feel the energy expand and contract.

7. When ready, move your palms back to your knees and keep breathing. Blow through your palms to remove the sensation.

Self-Treatments – Western Hand Positions

Some Western Reiki schools only place hands in certain positions on the body when giving a Reiki treatment, so I've included the basic positions and instructions on how to give yourself a self-treatment.

Before starting your self-treatment make sure the room is warm, as your temperature will drop as you relax into the treatment. Make sure you won't be disturbed – switch off your phone or tell others to give you some 'alone time'. Play some relaxing music. Take a seat or lie down, whichever you find the most comfortable.

Centre yourself, put your hands into Gassho (prayer position) and intend to give Reiki to yourself. Say a silent prayer to Usui, including any ancestors, gods, goddesses, angels and so on, or just the universe, asking to be a channel for Reiki to pass through you for the highest good of your own healing.

Intend that Reiki is coming from above and entering your

crown chakra, moving down your shoulders and along your arms and out through the palms of your hands. If you find it hard to focus, imagine that Reiki flows into your crown chakra as you breathe in, and flows out through the minor chakras in the palms of your hands as you breathe out. Whether you prefer Western or Eastern Reiki practices, you should always start from the top of your head, work down the body and finish on the soles of the feet. The general advice for Western hand positions is to leave your hands in each position for three to five minutes for a good cleansing, and the total treatment should last around 45 minutes.

I will, however, encourage you to tune in to your energy and stay in each position for as long as you feel you need to. You may find that on some areas of your body, your hands do not want to move or you feel a lot of tingling or heat. Keep your hands there for as long as your hands want to stay. Or you may find that your hands deflect off areas or there is a cold sensation; in that case, go to the sides of the cold spot or above it. Always feel with your hands and trust them. Don't think about where your hands should go; just trust that they are going to where they are needed.

If you feel nothing, that's not a problem and perfectly normal; just keep to the hand positions and focus on the intent. Sometimes we can't feel anything, but this probably means that the healing is working on a deeper level. Just remember to trust Reiki and that whatever is happening during a self-treatment, it is for your own highest good.

If you find that it is difficult to place your hands on any particular part of your body, just place your hands in a comfortable position on yourself like your lap or chest, and intend that Reiki will go to wherever it needs to. Try not to focus too much on timing and hand positions; let yourself relax and just let the Reiki flow.

I do advise that if you do the treatment at night before going to sleep (which is a great time to do it), try not to fall asleep during it. Also, if you find that you keep falling asleep during a self-treatment, it may suggest that you need grounding, which is discussed further in the manual.

Position 1: Place your hands over your eyes and forehead.

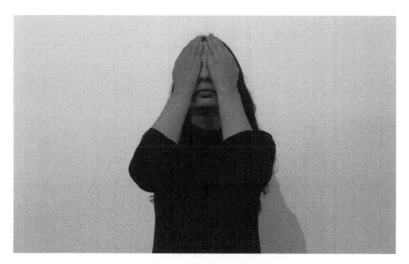

Position 1. Eyes and forehead

Position 2: Place your hands over your temples.

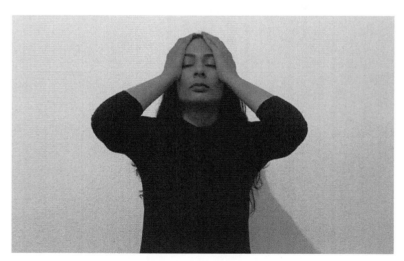

Position 2. Temples

Position 3: Place your hands over your ears.

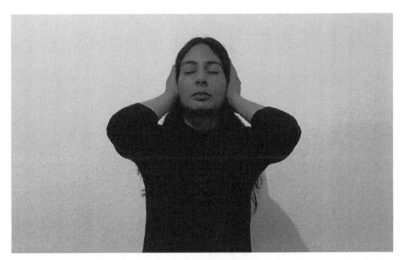

Position 3. Ears

Position 4: Place your hands over the base of your skull.

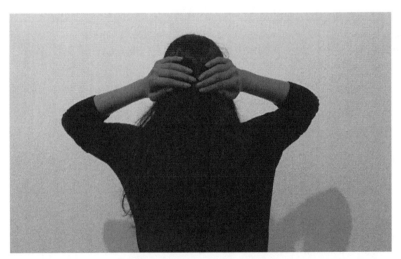

Position 4. Base of your skull

Position 5: Place your hands on your shoulders.

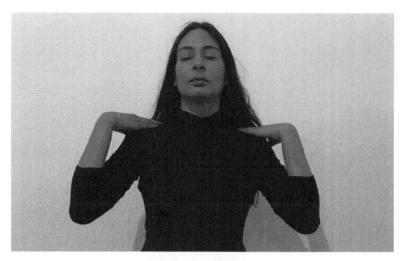

Position 5. Shoulders

Position 6: Place your hands on your throat chakra.

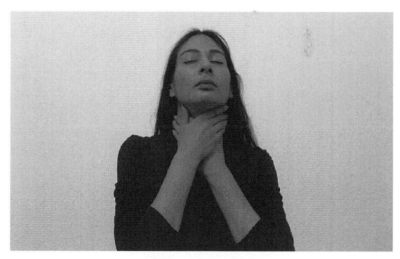

Position 6. Throat chakra

Position 7: Place your hands on your heart chakra.

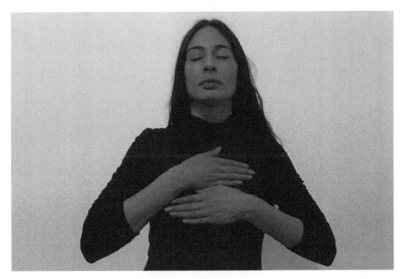

Position 7. Heart chakra

Position 8: Place your hands either side of your solar plexus.

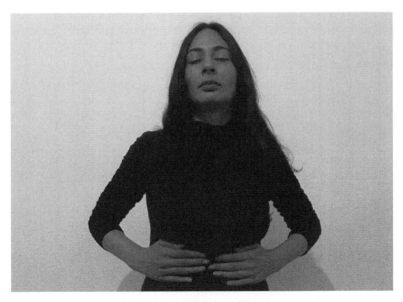

Position 8. Solar plexus

Position 9: Place your hands either side of your sacral chakra.

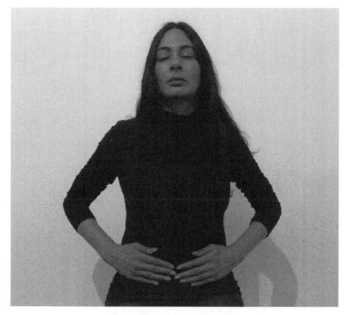

Position 9. Sacral chakra

Position 10: Place your hands either side of your root/base chakra covering your pelvis.

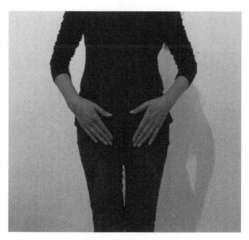

Position 10. Root chakra

Position 11: Place your hands onto the front of your knees.

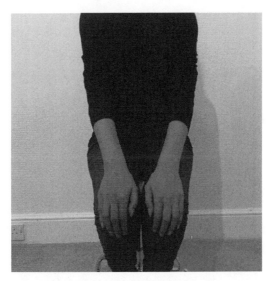

Position 11. Front of your knees

Position 12: Place your hands onto the back of your knees.

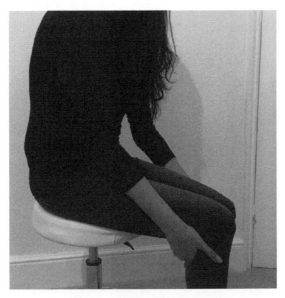

Position 12. Back of your knees

Position 13: Place one hand over the front of your ankle and the other over the back of your ankle.

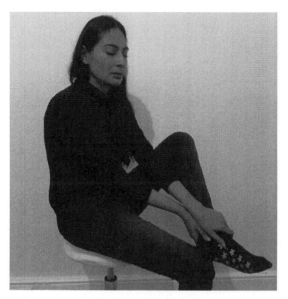

Position 13. First ankle

Position 14: Do the same on the other ankle.

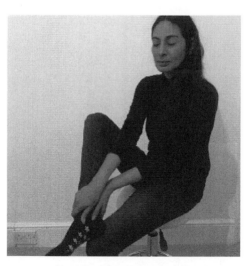

Position 14. Other ankle

Position 15: Place one hand on the top of your foot and the other on the sole.

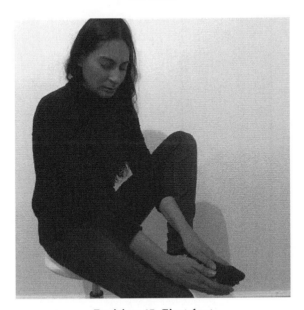

Position 15. First foot

Position 16: Do the same on the other foot.

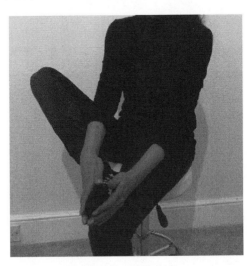

Position 16. Other foot

Position 17: Sweep your hands through your aura three times and then blow through your hands to clear away any lingering energy.

Position 18: Put your hands in Gassho and thank the universe for the Reiki healing.

If you're not comfortable with the Western hand positions, try the Japanese intuitive way which is covered further on.

I remember finding each 21-day Reiki cleanse really hard work and it even became a chore. This can be a normal thing for many Shoden students because it is hard work and it's easy to stop doing it. If you stop during the middle of a 21-day Reiki cleanse, don't worry; just start again from the beginning and sometimes just limit the treatment to ten minutes. Self-treatments should be considered a time for self-love, for healing and taking care of yourself, but at times it can be uncomfortable and hard to complete.

I now find it really easy to give myself Reiki treatments and do so on a very regular basis. However, when I have something I want to focus on like an illness or feeling out of sorts, I commit to a 21-day Reiki cleanse for that particular issue and I'm in a space where I enjoy them and see them as 'me time'.

Japanese Philosophies and Practice of Original Usui Reiki

The Original Japanese Usui Reiki practices became known to Western Practitioners in the 1990s when Usui's original texts and students were discovered in Japan. Many Reiki Practitioners have now combined both Western and Original Japanese Usui Reiki practices to suit themselves. Having the information and being able to practise both philosophies allows you to combine and use what comes more naturally to you. There is no right or wrong way. Reiki healing not only works for your highest good; I think that Reiki practice also developed and adapted globally according to how we as human beings needed it.

Original Japanese Usui Reiki has its own rituals performed at the beginning and end of treatments, and the treatments themselves are very much based on trusting your intuition and scanning the energy field. Usui's teachings were intense and his students met weekly to meditate, apply Reiki together and practise scanning the body until they succeeded in reaching a type of energetic diagnosis. They would then treat those areas of the body and it was very specific and precise work.

The main difference in practising Reiki from the Western to Japanese perspective is that in the West, more emphasis is put on the hand positions. In Japanese Usui Reiki the emphasis is to ensure that the Reiki treatment starts on the head and finishes with the feet; the middle part is all about feeling the energy and trusting Reiki to show you where to put your hands. Usui's teachings stated that plenty of time is required to be spent on the head and on the feet, and in Japan a Reiki treatment can last up to two hours and beyond.

Reiki practice in the East is seen as personal development, which takes time to process and learn, whereas in the West it developed more quickly with less time spent between the Degrees. However, life now in Japan and the Eastern world is also moving at a much faster pace and fewer people in general around the world take time to heal. Time is seen as precious, but it's important to remember that healing takes time, practice and patience. The old saying, 'Healer, heal thyself', is important for Reiki Practitioners to remember in order to spend time healing, connecting and getting to know their own unique relationship with Reiki.

In Japan, where spirituality lies in a mixture of Shinto (the belief that every living creature or objects such as rocks, trees, rivers and mountains all have their own spirits) and Zen Buddhism, karma is deemed important for the soul path, and reincarnation is part and parcel of many Eastern spiritual paths. Generally, Western views are very much based on this lifetime or a soul that does not reincarnate. Both viewpoints are important. Whether you believe in reincarnation or not doesn't really matter, so long as you are aware of your personal life force, energy field, aura, soul, spirit, or you may call it your 'essence'.

In the West many people wouldn't consider that an illness could be brought into their life as a soul lesson – that there is a reason for the illness, that a life lesson must be taught, that changes must be made on a mental/emotional/soul level before a physical issue can be cured, or that the physical illness may actually be a result of karma from a different lifetime. This is very much an Eastern viewpoint of dis-ease, but dis-ease may also be brought into our lives by trauma we have faced in this lifetime. So, when giving Reiki healing, it is important to not make assumptions but to just let the healing take place at its own pace.

In Japan there are other types of energy healing practices using the hands, but it seems that Usui Reiki is the most popular. It had the opportunity to travel around the world, change, adapt and then be reintroduced back to Japan from the West, only for the original Usui rituals to be bought forward by his students and come to the West.

The Five Principles of Reiki

The emperor Meiji over his lifetime wrote thousands of Waka poems and was famous for them. He originally wrote the Waka poems which Usui adopted into 'The Five Principles of Reiki'. Usui used 125 Waka poems in total for Reiki healing to encourage his students to live a meaningful, wholesome life. He knew the importance of positive, disciplined thinking and how a healthy mindset can change your life for the better. The Five Principles of Reiki are:

Just for today:
Do not get angry
Do not worry
Be grateful
Do your duties fully
Be kind to others

When I was first taught the Five Principles, I was actually taught slightly different wording and for some reason I didn't connect with them. It is strange how simple words or sentences can cause you to overthink. I found that I questioned if I was worthy enough to actually live by them, and if I actually wanted to live by them. They have at times left me feeling slightly guilty about things I've done, and I've had to learn to find my own path with them. So do not overthink them. The Five Principles are an extremely useful tool for practising mindfulness and to live a more wholesome lifestyle, but you have to be able to bring them into your heart if you want to really learn from them.

The Five Principles of Reiki are as follows in both English and Japanese, and below, I have described what the principles mean to me personally. You will find different versions when researching them.

Just for today – *Kyo dake wa*

'Just for today' is about coming into the present moment to focus on each of the Five Principles individually and remember that I have the ability to choose how I react or respond. I can plan for tomorrow and I can learn lessons from yesterday, but it is only in this moment that I have the ability to live, to breathe, to love, to really be alive and fully experience everything that is going on around me or inside me. It is a reminder that just for today, I can be free from anger and worry, and I can focus on being grateful, doing my duties fully and being kind.

Now this is a strange one, but because I am a procrastinator,

I can find it difficult to think of 'just for today'. In many ways, I am happy today and I can focus on that, but getting stuff done is at times very hard for me. I have to make daily lists to ensure that I don't put things off, but I get very anxious about getting things done. It's like a fear of completing things. So I focus on what I can do now and sometimes I let that be just getting the little things done like washing the dishes. I do actually reward myself for completing tasks now, whilst I can, and I do always feel so much better once I've finished something. Yes, 'just for today' can leave knots in the pit of my stomach, but I am aware of this and I try to be kind to myself and find a way to work with myself to avoid the anxiety.

Do not get angry – *Ikaru na*

This allows me to practise calm, to try to find peace in the midst of despair. I've found that since reciting the Five Principles to myself, I have learned how to stand back and observe situations, make sense of them and understand why I feel anger. Reciting 'Just for today, do not get angry' like a mantra allows me to respond to situations or people with calm, clarity and standing firm with what I believe in. I can now feel more confident communicating from my heart without getting frustrated or stuck.

Anger can be a very healthy emotion and it is important to listen to your anger, to learn what has caused it and understand why you feel it. To suppress anger only drives it deeper within you and this can cause dis-ease. Being able to take responsibility for your anger enables you to use it to change your life for the better, in dealing with situations or with relationships. Understanding and dealing with anger is an important step to healing.

Do not worry – *Shin pai suna*

Learning to not worry is probably one of the hardest things to have to do in life. It is also something that I have had to relearn over and over again. To let go of worry is, I think, something that is much harder to do when loved ones are involved, but the truth is that there is no point in worrying about things you cannot control. Worry brings about fear, which if focused on can have damaging negative effects on our well-being. To be able to let go of worry, and to think about positive outcomes and not negative ones, can spur us on to do great things. It is something that requires a lot of practice, but reminding yourself that in this moment there is no point in worrying really does help.

Worry can be a positive emotion. It can challenge you to change things, to take control and let go of the things that cause your worry. There's trust in not worrying, and that comes from inner peace.

Be grateful – *Kan sha shi te*

Now this one has caught me out many a time. There have been plenty of times when gratefulness has gone completely out of the window to be replaced with ungratefulness. I try to remind myself that just for today I am grateful for waking up on this morning. I am grateful for my partner, my family and friends, a roof over my head and food in my belly. I believe positivity attracts positivity, so I try to see problems and complications as character building, as growth, as an opportunity to overcome and succeed. I'm grateful to the universe for all the little things that make me smile today. Yes, I do still get days when I want to slap the universe and hide under a duvet, and to be honest, I'm grateful I can do that once in a while. I think being grateful reminds us of what is important; it allows us to smile and gives us joy, and that is a positive thing.

Do your duties fully – *Gyo-o hage me*

The wording of this principle can be kind of daunting. Duties…

What if your boss or family think that your duty is something that *you* feel you're being pressured into? That you 'doing your duty' is living a life that you're not happy in? Well, then you're not doing your duty to yourself. It could mean spiritual duty, social duty, family duty, work duty, environmental duty or cultural duty. I personally think that we need to be honest with ourselves and follow what feels right in our hearts. Reiki is for the self, first and foremost, and we should put our duties to ourselves first without hurting others, with the realisation that there is give and take in every situation. Be honest with yourself. I think that is the best way for me, anyhow, to do my duties fully.

Be kind to others – *Hito ni shin setsu ni*

Really, this should be the first and most important law in every country. How different our lives would be if people really practised being kind to each other, to Mother Earth and the creatures of our lands, seas and skies. To ourselves. This is about being able to recognise and honour the divine in everyone and within ourselves. Being kind really does lead to a more peaceful existence.

Usui recognised how people, regardless of any healing they had, would never evolve if their mindsets were stuck in the same cycles. The Five Principles of Reiki were developed by Usui to guide people to recognise their own thought patterns and encourage the discipline to change behaviour patterns. If you continually keep thinking, *Life is hard*, or *I'm not happy with my body or my situation*, or *No one likes me*, or *I will only be happy when such and such happens*, you are never going to evolve. You will never be happy or content, because these basic requirements for a healthy, happy mind come from within and not from material objects or others' approval.

Cultivating a healthy mindset and thought patterns

41

encourages you to observe and deal with stress and trauma in a mindful, wholesome and more positive manner. Trauma of some kind or other is the reason why most of my clients come for Reiki treatments. People hold on to trauma; we shield it from others, protect it and can't let go of the crushing negative feelings because sometimes we don't know who we are without them. Even when we are at our most fragile, pride and ego can keep us in the trauma and it's incredibly hard to let go of, because it's our reality and has become such a big part of us.

Keeping the Five Principles close to your heart and repeating them really does encourage you to strive, to take any benefit from the trauma, and then let the trauma go. Understanding them and using them to live a better life for yourself and others brings peace and contentment. It can take a while but it's worth it.

With each thought that we have, we produce positive or negative energy vibrations. When we are thinking something negative about ourselves, we are attacking ourselves, and in turn, anything we send out will ultimately affect the people around us, and our environment. It is extremely easy when we are hurt or angry, or when we fear something, to project this negativity out onto others and deeper within ourselves. Even when we love someone and wouldn't physically hurt them, it is easy to project our fears, anger and hurt onto them and unintentionally attack them with our negative thoughts.

When we are focused on trying to send out positivity, regardless of how hard it can be at times, we are sending out love and healing. When we can give ourselves a big hug and really try to give ourselves a little love, it in turn is sent out to all around us.

Regardless of how blessed our lives may be today, we cannot control external or even internal factors, such as sudden illness, accidents, economic factors, or even the weather. The one thing we can control – learn to control – is how we react to situations.

We can learn to turn negatives into positives, to see that the glass is not just half full – it's refillable, or maybe we can just pick another drink instead. To basically see the potential in every situation.

Reciting the Five Principles to yourself is a great reminder of how to remain grounded and allows you to see the opportunities in each negative situation. Staying true to yourself, giving yourself Reiki for your highest good, cleansing and removing any negativity, allows you to find your highest potential.

Practising the Five Principles of Reiki

Many Reiki Practitioners will frame and display the Five Principles of Reiki in the room where they practise Reiki. It is important to not let the Five Principles of Reiki disappear into the background but to really make them a part of your life.

Start your day by reciting the Five Principles. Place your hands in Gassho and recite them mindfully. Think about the meaning of them and how they reflect your life. Meditate with them; chanting them like a mantra will help you focus. If you're having a particularly bad day, focus on the one that you need. Practice makes it easier to become detached from whatever is no longer serving you for your highest good.

Many Reiki Practitioners recite the Five Principles before and after giving a Reiki treatment as they encourage you to focus on the healing and be in a space of love.

Breath

In all esoteric traditions, breath is the bridge between the body and consciousness. During meditations or yoga and such like, learned breathing is considered vital for taking into your body the energy of life and releasing negativity back out.

When I meditate, I find that focusing on my breathing at the start enables me to stay in the moment with more ease, allows me to feel calm and basically enhances my meditations. It also helps with focusing when giving Reiki treatments. It can take some practising, as we normally only breathe through our nose, but this does allow us to focus on the life force which we are taking into our body, mind, heart and soul, and to release any negativity which no longer serves us.

- Inhale through your nose with your tongue resting on the roof of your mouth.
- Exhale through your mouth with your tongue at the bottom of your mouth.
- Continue as above.

Gassho Meiso

The Japanese word *Gassho* translates into 'two hands coming together' and *Meiso* translates to 'meditation'. This is the normal prayer position where your hands come together in front of your chest. It is the preparation for meditation and is basically about focus. Focusing on your two middle fingers focuses the mind. When practising Gassho Meiso, you may find that your hands start to heat up, but you must remember to keep focused.

To practise Gassho Meiso, follow the steps below:

1. Close your eyes and be in a relaxed position, either lying down or sitting on a chair. If sitting, keep your back as straight as possible without straining it; use a cushion if required.
2. Bring both hands together comfortably in front of your heart chakra.
3. Breathe.
4. Focus your attention on the point where the two middle fingers meet.
5. If your hands become tired during the meditation, allow them to rest in your lap, keeping the attention on the middle fingers.

Hat Su Rei Ho

Hat Su is literally translated into 'generate', *Rei* into 'universal' and *Ho* into 'method/technique', but the meaning translates as 'start up Reiki technique'. When practising Hat Su Rei Ho, you should find that this meditation enhances the flow of the energy when giving a treatment, as well as cleansing the self and enhancing the conscious channelling of energy.

Usui's students practised Hat Su Rei Ho on a daily basis, as well as the Five Principles, and they also received regular Reiju Empowerments. It was taught that daily practice of Hat Su Rei Ho, combined with daily treatments and regular use of Reiki, encouraged development of your intuition and spiritual awareness.

Stage 1 – Relax:

Close your eyes, place hands on your lap and concentrate on using your breath to bring presence into your body. Focus on your *dantien* point (two fingers below your navel and a third of the way in).

Stage 2 – Mokunen (Focusing):

Set the intention and say to yourself, 'I am going to start Hat Su Rei Ho.'

Stage 3 – Kenyoko (Dry brushing):

Kenyoko is used to brush off negative energy. You can use it before or after Reiki or at any point where you feel you need to refresh and centre:

1. Whilst inhaling, place the fingertips of your right hand at the top of your left shoulder with your hand lying flat against your chest.
2. As you exhale, making a 'haaaa' sound, sweep your hand lightly and smoothly down your body diagonally,

arriving at your right hip.

3. Whilst inhaling, place the fingertips of your left hand at the top of your right shoulder with your hand lying flat against your chest.

4. As you exhale, making a 'haaaa' sound, sweep your hand lightly and smoothly down your body diagonally, arriving at your left hip.

5. Repeat steps 1 to 4.

6. Now whilst inhaling, place your right fingertips onto the outer edge of your left shoulder and slightly outstretch your arm so your hand is not flat on your chest.

7. As you exhale, making a 'haaaa' sound, sweep your hand lightly and smoothly down your body diagonally, arriving at your right hip.

8. Inhale and place your left fingertips onto the outer edge of your right shoulder and slightly outstretch your arm so your hand is not flat on your chest.

9. As you exhale, making a 'haaaa' sound, sweep your hand lightly and smoothly down your body diagonally, arriving at your right hip.

10. Repeat steps 6 to 9.

Stage 4 – Joshin Kokkyu Ho (Technique for purification of spirit):

1. Put your hands in your lap, palms facing upwards, breathing naturally through your nose if you can.

2. As you inhale, visualise white light flooding into your crown chakra and palms, and filling your dantien.

3. Feel it gather there as you pause.

4. Exhale, intending that the light floods out of you, stretching out into infinity.

5. Continue to add to the energy by repeating the above for several minutes.

Stage 5 – Gassho:

Bringing your hands together in Gassho, hold this position, focusing on your middle fingers for the rest of the meditation.

Stage 6 – Seishin Toitsu (Continued meditation):

1. Stay in Gassho.
2. As you inhale, visualise white light flooding from your hands into your heart chakra.
3. As you exhale, visualise the white light flooding from your heart chakra into your hands.
4. Repeat steps 2 and 3 for several minutes.
5. Before finishing, you may wish to repeat the Five Principles to yourself.
6. To finish, part your hands whilst saying to yourself that you have now finished Hat Su Rei Ho. Disconnect or continue into a treatment.

Reiji Ho

Reiji translates to 'indication of spirit' and *Ho* is 'method', so this ritual teaches us to follow our intuition. This is a method of not only trusting the universe to guide you in the healing of yourself or another but also trusting your own instincts. It allows you to stop using your brain as such and to go on 'feeling'.

This is something I do before every Reiki treatment, be it for myself or a client, and so I've worded the following for both.

1. Sit or stand in a comfortable position and close your eyes. (I normally do this standing up by the client's head just before starting a treatment.)
2. Hold your hands in Gassho and ask Reiki to flow through you freely. (You should feel the Reiki flow through you, either by entering your crown chakra, or as warmth in your heart area or in your hands. Each person

is different, so you will feel Reiki flow into you in your own way.)

3. Ask for the healing (of yourself or a client) to be on every level (emotional, mental, physical or energetic) and dedicate it for the highest good.

4. Raise your hands in the Gassho position to your third eye and ask that your hands be a tool for Reiki and be guided to where they need to be.

Now you wait and see what happens, but most importantly, follow your first instinct even if it doesn't make sense. No matter how big or small your instinct, remember it may be known to you in many ways, such as a pull to a certain area, an inner knowing, seeing the area that needs healing, or even hearing it.

Byosen

Byo translates into 'ill or toxic' and *sen* translates into 'lump', so Byosen translates into 'lump of toxins'. I have also been told that Byosen translates into 'sick line', but the basic meaning is the same.

Using Byosen, we can scan the body to find the area where the lump of toxins or the sick line is. The most common areas for the toxins to accumulate tend to be in and around the kidneys and joints like the upper back, armpits, shoulders and neck.

I don't know why, but I find it's easier to feel Byosen when treating others, so I've worded the following as if treating a client. We start with Reiji Ho, by asking for guidance, then try to scan the recipient's body with our hands. You should start to feel sensations, but if you at first find it difficult to sense anything, try the following:

- Stand to the side of the recipient and place your dominant hand on or above their crown chakra and attune yourself to it.

- If you still don't feel guided, run your hand slowly along their *hara* line, which runs down the centre of the body.

Byosen has different levels that can be identified as below.

Level 1. On-Netsu (Warmth):
You should be able to sense warmth with your hands over areas of the recipient's body which have negativity, energy blocks or dis-ease.

Level 2. Atsui-On-Netsu (Intense heat):
The warmth will be followed by intense heat felt in your palms.

Level 3. Piri-Piri Kan (Tingling sensation):
If the negativity, blockage or dis-ease level is quite high, you will feel a tingling sensation in your palms or fingertips. Some describe this sensation as electric vibration or numbness.

Level 4. Hibiki (Throbbing sensation):
This is a pulse-like sensation in your hands, which indicates that you can actually feel Reiki stimulating the blood vessels, causing them to expand and contract, thus improving the circulation of the blood flow.

Level 5. Itami (Pain):
If the Byosen is quite serious you can feel pain in your hands, which can spread up your arm to your elbows. You may also feel a lot of tingling. Do not be alarmed if you feel any pain; it will disappear as the Reiki works, and you must always remember that, as the Reiki Practitioner, you are protected.

When I first started to do energy healing, I used to see people in an X-ray kind of way and the problem areas were shown up like an X-ray. That's changed for me as now I tend to focus more on feeling, so I trust Byosen and let it lead me. My hands tend to feel heat or the tingling sensation whilst doing the Reiji Ho, and then when I scan the body, I can feel the different ranges of heat, tingling and throbbing, or my hands feel as if they are being pulled by energy to where they need to go. The main thing is that you just need to trust your instinct and practice. If you find that you don't feel any Byosen, stick to the hand positions taught in Western Reiki.

I should also mention that you may feel or experience other things during a Reiki treatment, such as your stomach rumbling, a cough, feeling tearful, or actual pain where the client is feeling it. These all pass after a few minutes.

Other Japanese Techniques

A typical Japanese treatment always starts with giving Reiki to the head first, regardless of symptoms, because the basic nature of Reiki flows from the head to the feet. Always feel for Byosen on the head first, then the body, and finish the treatment on the soles of the feet. It is said that you should spend at least 30 minutes on the head, but I think it best to use your intuition and trust in Byosen and your hands. However, as Reiki is always working for the highest good of the person being treated, it will go to wherever it is needed.

One Japanese school states that Usui received Reiki energy with his left hand and passed it on to his right hand. He is said to have brought the fingertips of his left hand together with his thumb. With his right hand, he would touch the fingertips of his middle and ring fingers with his thumb. His little finger and index finger were said to have stood away from the other fingers at a 90-degree angle. This is supposed to create a laser-like beam which focuses on a small area of the body.

Usui was also known to use a series of techniques in which he used touch, massage, stroking, blowing, staring and tapping onto areas of the body. The more time you spend practising

Reiki, the more you trust what techniques work for you. I do have a client who I massage and stroke whilst giving Reiki to them, but that really is something the client and I are comfortable with, and I let my hands and fingers do what they feel is needed for the client. I also find that sometimes I release Reiki from my third eye as well as my hands, and sometimes I stare at the problem area and Reiki is released through my eyes. Before tapping, stroking, massaging or staring at a client, check with them first to ensure that they don't mind.

Though Reiki is deemed to be about spiritual development, Usui was very much interested in distortions of the spine and the spinal vertebrae, and studied how issues with the spine can affect the health of a person. He used Reiki to help heal issues with the spine to remove dis-ease, whereas Dr Hayashi, who had a medical background, was very much interested in how Reiki healed the body's major organs. In Japan, focusing only on the physical body does not take away from the spiritual aspect of healing, as science and spirit are deemed to be 'one'.

Other Reiki Treatments

Treating animals

Animals are very receptive to Reiki and if you have a pet, you may sense a change in their reaction to you when you've been attuned: they can't get enough of you or they run off whenever you're near them. If you want to give your pet Reiki, they will usually let you know if they want it or not. If they don't, they will just walk off. If they do want it, just let your hands lie down on them and they will actually move around if they feel it is needed in certain areas. If you want to do Reiki on their chakras, remember that their chakras tend to be aligned just the same as in humans.

I used to have a dog client called Mia. She had multiple heath issues and she loved Reiki. Whenever she saw me, she would jump onto me at the front door and put whatever part of her body that needed Reiki into my hands. Most of the time it was her rear end. As soon as I put on my Reiki music, she would get onto her bed and wait for me to start the treatment. She knew she was receiving Reiki and she would lie there and lap it up.

Be aware that some animals will not react to Reiki and some may reject it. As with humans, we don't force Reiki on anyone, so if an animal rejects it, don't try to push it. They will accept it when they are ready.

Treating plants

Now plants can't run off if they don't want Reiki, but if they do want it, you may actually feel a tingling or heat in your palms whenever you are around them. The best thing to do is to tune in to the plant's energy and feel Reiki being drawn into them. I give all my plants Reiki, and some of my smaller or new plants receive Reiki on a regular basis. I'm not a green-fingered person, and to grow and care for my plants I tend to google a lot. But I have found that giving them Reiki does encourage their well-being. I do treat my plants like they are family because I love them, and I think that is important too.

Treating food and drink

Reiki can be used to raise the vibration of food and drink and it is a positive thing to do before a meal – much like a blessing before having a meal. There have been experiments conducted on using Reiki to raise the vibration of water, which resulted in positive effects on the person who consumes it.

Mr Masaru Emoto discovered that by praising water, the water formed into beautiful crystals which could be seen under a microscope. When the water was spoken to in a harsh way, the crystals became malformed and fragmented. Energy vibrations are in everything, from the air to water to humans, and when treated in a positive way, the energy vibrations rise. So by giving

Reiki to our food and drink, we raise the vibrational energy of what we are about to consume and take into our body.

Treating negativity

Reiki can be used to clear negativity from a house, an object or even an interaction. I use Reiki to cleanse my crystals, my laptop and even my home. When cleansing my home, I place my palms in front of me and allow the Reiki to flow into my crown chakra, down my arms and through my palms into the space that I want cleansed. I visualise the energy spreading out into the space and filling up all the dark corners.

I always use Reiki when dealing with negativity from interactions, and recite the Five Principles of Reiki to myself. I see no point in allowing others' interactions to leave negative energy around me, not any more. I clear it and I walk away.

Working with crystals

Working with crystals can be extremely beneficial as they not only have their own healing properties but can also be used to help cleanse your chakras, and aid physical, mental and emotional trauma. Crystals can also be used to heal or rebalance anything electrical, including computers, or even a space like a house. When choosing crystals always pick the stone that is speaking to you and do not pick crystals just because they are the biggest or the prettiest. There is a belief that, much like Reiki choosing you, crystals also choose you.

For a Reiki treatment, the crystals most commonly used for rebalancing and cleansing chakras are as follows, but I would recommend researching more on crystal energy and their healing properties.

- Root/base chakra – garnet, black tourmaline, onyx or smoky quartz
- Sacral chakra – carnelian or orange fire agate

- Solar plexus chakra – citrine
- Heart chakra – rose quartz, green tourmaline, aventurine or green garnet
- Throat chakra – aquamarine, turquoise, lapis lazuli, sodalite or angelate
- Third eye chakra – amethyst or quartz
- Crown chakra – quartz

I have a decent collection of crystals and I let my clients choose whichever crystals are drawn to them. After the Reiki treatment, we look up the meaning and healing properties of their chosen crystals to see how these relate to what healing they were after. It still surprises me how the crystals tend to be exactly what they need.

I always cleanse my crystals before and after a treatment with Reiki. It is very simple; just place the crystal in your palms, open up to the Reiki energy, feel it enter your crown chakra, through your arms into your palms, and visualise the energy pouring into the object and cleansing it. I also always leave crystals out during a new or full moon, so they can receive moon energy cleansing.

Clairvoyant practice

Now, for those who have never felt spirit around them, be aware that once attuned, Reiki can turn on or turn up your clairvoyance skills. You may find when doing a Reiki treatment that spiritual entities (guides, ancestors, angels and so on) may decide to come and join you. Do not be alarmed by this if you have never been in a similar situation. If it does happen and you are uncomfortable, ask the entities to hide themselves from you. I know this may sound a bit far-fetched. But I do believe that sometimes entities also join in with healing, and for me it is all about universal love. So it's a great thing. If, however, you are finding it difficult, remember you can stop and take a moment to yourself. Shut down that part of you and start again.

I had a client once who was new to Reiki and wasn't necessarily spiritual. She was just looking for a relaxing Reiki treatment, but from the start of the treatment to the end she felt hands on her shoulders and just accepted that they were there, though she knew I was touching another part of her body. It surprised her, but she liked the warmth that she was feeling and she didn't know what it was, only that someone else's hands had joined in with the healing. This can scare some people, but I always find it beautiful when others join in on a treatment. I didn't sense the hands at all, and sometimes I don't. You never really know what to expect in a treatment.

An important thing to consider if you do have a clairvoyant experience during a Reiki treatment for another person is whether to discuss it with them or not. It really depends on them and how open they are to receiving information from the universe. If there is a message, do you tell them? Well, if there is a message it may be that it is for their highest good to know; maybe they received the message too but think it may be just in their mind… I personally think that if they are open to receiving messages, you should tell them, but if they are not, then the universe will find a way to show them. What you can't do is think you know what is best for them. A lot of people don't believe in spirit and are uncomfortable with receiving messages. If a client asks for your feedback after a Reiki treatment, you need to judge whether they are open to receiving messages.

General Guidance for Shoden 1st Degree Level

The true focus of Reiki is our own well-being and spiritual development, and particularly in Shoden 1st Degree the emphasis really has to be on healing the self, first and foremost. However, we can be a channel for others' healing too, though professional practice of Reiki is not permitted until you have completed the Okuden 2nd Degree. It should also be noted that most Reiki Masters prefer that you take a minimum of six months between each Degree as this allows enough time for the cleansing period.

You do not need to take the Okuden 2nd Degree or Shihan Master Degree to have a better connection. Those Degrees are different because you learn to work with different energies, so never feel that your 1st Degree is not good enough. People work with Reiki for all sorts of reasons and I feel it's best to work with the Reiki energy until you feel a need to learn more. Do your own research. Find your own foundations with Reiki. Feel it and use it and take your time to get to know it. Trust that Reiki will always work for your highest good.

Intention

Intention is key to Reiki healing, and without intent, symbols and Kotodama, just the act of giving Reiki does not work. If the intention is not the focus, then there is no focus in Reiki healing.

When Usui taught his students the different Kotodama and symbols to connect to the different energies of Reiki, it was so that once used to the method of connecting to the different frequencies, intent would be all that you need. Experienced Reiki Masters find that sooner or later the symbols do actually take a step back, because 'intention' is the only thing required to connect to the different energy frequencies of Reiki.

Ethics

This is for Reiki Practitioners but good for those at Shoden level to be aware of. Reiki is by no means a substitute for modern medicine, and legally a Reiki Practitioner must recommend a GP or medical professional if there is a requirement. Never diagnose an illness or tell a client you can heal their medical condition. Not only is it illegal and misguiding; it's also not morally right to give false hope.

As healers, we never force Reiki on anyone, especially if they don't want it. When people want Reiki they will come to you. There is nothing wrong with letting people know that you now have the Shoden 1st Degree, but pushing people into receiving treatments is considered unethical in the Reiki world. The people you give Reiki to need to be comfortable with you, and that will come from them having made the choice to have a treatment from you. They will come to you or go elsewhere when they are ready to receive treatments, and we as healers must honour that and trust in our own Reiki journey. Reiki will bring to you those you are meant to be in contact with at the right time for you both.

It is also important to remember that if anybody is trying to press you into giving them a treatment and you're not comfortable with it, say no. You have to trust in your intuition.

Energy exchange

It is important that an energy exchange is conducted when giving Reiki treatments. I don't think this is so important when dealing with loved ones, as these relationships are based on love and so energy is constantly exchanged. I've done many Reiki treatments on friends and we've exchanged energy via a home-cooked meal, or in one case a friend who is a massage therapist gave me a massage and then I gave her Reiki. So we constantly exchanged energy.

However, after the Okuden 2nd Degree and becoming a professional Reiki Practitioner, a professional exchange should take place with the client. Reiki not only needs value put on it, but also if a Reiki Practitioner is constantly giving out free energy, their energy can begin to dry up and result in burnout. Never let anyone push you into giving Reiki for free. If they're having money problems and you feel a need to give them Reiki treatment, then ensure that some other sort of exchange is made.

Detachment

As healers, we need to practise detachment when giving Reiki treatments to ourselves and others, and it is good to remember we are but a channel for Reiki. To get involved mentally or emotionally with your healing or the healing of others can have negative effects in the long run. Yes, detachment from your own healing is achievable. It's all about trust. The outcome will be the outcome. All you can do is trust and believe that Reiki is working for the highest good of the person being treated.

Protection

During Reiki treatments, picking up vibes from the client is commonplace and a Practitioner may feel some of the client's issues, for example a painful elbow, or a need to cry. However, as the Reiki is going through you to the recipient, you are protected from their energy. So if you feel anything unusual, do not be alarmed. It normally disappears after a few minutes. Nevertheless, to ensure that you are protected from any blocked or negative energy, follow these guidelines:

1. Never treat anyone you don't want to. If you get bad vibes or feel uncomfortable, say no to the treatment.
2. Always ensure there is an equal energy exchange.
3. Always cleanse yourself after a treatment by blowing away any leftover energy, washing down your hands, and giving yourself a quick Reiki cleanse.

Resistance you may face for being a healer

As a healer, you may come across people with very different viewpoints from you and many judgements, but it is important to remember that you are on your Reiki journey and each person you meet will be a part of your healing process. Reiki healing is becoming more mainstream and can now be found being used within the health and care services. I believe this will bring more people to the benefits of Reiki healing, whether they use it just for relaxation and general well-being, to heal emotional, mental or physical trauma, or as a spiritual gift. But there is still a lot of negativity towards energy healing practices, and any negativity you receive should be seen as an opportunity to grow, to learn how to deal with negativity and to be more receptive to healing.

I've lost clients in the past due to pressure they were put under from people they knew. One in particular was confronted by a church member who was convinced Reiki is the devil's work. The client only had one treatment and never came back, and yes, I was offended by the idea that people really believe that energy healing is only 'good' if it is given by a member of a particular religion. Energy healing is still energy healing, regardless of who is doing it, or which path or method we use.

There have also been times when people have questioned the science of Reiki, thus trying to show that it's not scientifically proven and therefore it doesn't exist. I've always found that those who make this argument are as closed-minded as the people who believe it to be the devil's work. I believe it's like arguing that oxygen doesn't exist because we can't see it.

But all of this negativity can be a positive thing, because it makes me realise all the more how different people, cultures, lives are, and how there is beauty in all the differences. It is rewarding to have an open dialogue and conversation about healing, because we can learn so much from others and find some connection between us.

Different effects of Reiki treatments

This is something that I find a lot of people are unaware of. Reiki treatments are not always lovely, relaxing or comforting. Having a Reiki treatment can be uncomfortable, even painful, and leave you crying for days on end.

Reiki will cleanse you for your own highest good and will go to where it is needed, regardless of what you think you want or need. However, we need to be careful of how others are feeling when we give them a Reiki treatment.

With a physical problem, for example a painful pulled muscle or nerve tension, it is really important to let clients know that they must move if they are uncomfortable. I've had clients in the past who were very uncomfortable but didn't want to say, so they ended up feeling worse than when they came for the treatment. So it's a good idea to keep an eye on them to ensure that they are not in pain or uncomfortable. Reassure them that if they need to change their position, they can do so.

Reiki treatments can also be very uncomfortable emotionally and mentally. Whilst I was in the Middle East, I had a Reiki treatment by a Reiki Master and it felt as if I had tiny ants crawling under my skin for the entire treatment. I lay there just wanting it to end, to stop the feeling that was freaking me out. It was so uncomfortable but it was what I needed. I was letting go of so much trauma whilst there, and that one treatment represented, in a way, the negativity being cleansed out of my system.

I've also had clients who seemed almost ashamed for becoming emotional during a Reiki treatment, but it is so important to let these emotions out, to cry if the need takes place. There is no shame in feeling sad. It's only a shame if one can't let the sadness pass.

So whilst most Reiki treatments are lovely and relaxing and nice, it is good to be aware of how uncomfortable they can also be.

If you stop practising Reiki

If you continue to practise Reiki, remember that the more you channel Reiki, the better the flow. However, if you stop channelling Reiki, you will find that it is harder to reconnect, though you will not lose your ability. If you find that you haven't channelled Reiki for a while, and are finding it hard to reconnect, just keep practising and remember that intention is key. Try it for five minutes and work your way up to a full-body treatment. Don't try to force it. Just give yourself a little time to focus. You can, however, always get yourself attuned again.

Chapter 2

Okuden 2nd Degree of Original Usui Reiki

Eastern and Western Philosophies

Introduction

On the Okuden 2nd Degree, the Attunements and Reiju Empowerments that are given connect you to two different healing-energy frequencies which cleanse and heal on deeper levels. You are given the tools – the symbols and Kotodama – to identify and use these two different energy frequencies, and learn how to build a cosmic bridge to send Reiki over space and time. Though most Reiki 1st Degree students are taught how to give Reiki to others, having the Okuden Degree gives you the opportunity to be a professional Reiki Practitioner and practise Reiki within the limits of the law. So I've included the basics of how to give professional Reiki treatments.

Healing should be universal and everyone has the ability to heal; however, being a professional Reiki Practitioner is about trust, and with this trust comes responsibility and respect. When we are attuned to Reiki, we are activated to particular energy frequencies and we become a channel for these energy frequencies.

However, being a Reiki Practitioner is much more than being a channel for Reiki. As a professional Reiki Practitioner, your clients will come to you with the expectation that their healing is sacred, is private, and you are in a position of responsibility. You are the person they have come to for help in healing their trauma, their dis-ease, and they have put their trust in you. This above all else should be honoured.

The Okuden Cleansing

The Attunements and/or Reiju Empowerments on Okuden are aimed at connecting you to the different energy frequencies which heal on the deeper emotional, mental and spiritual levels and work mainly on the throat, heart and third eye chakras. Common experiences of this level of cleansing are:

- Throat – a releasing of unspoken or repressed emotions and being able to communicate more effectively and truthfully with yourself or others. This may be accompanied by physical throat ailments.
- Heart – there may be an arising of emotions or past hurts, some of which you may not have even been aware of. You may find yourself grieving over a past situation or loss that you thought you had already grieved over, or one that you didn't want to give time to before. You may become very emotional and not know why – feeling things more deeply, passionately and in a more connected way. Physically this could be felt as ailments of the heart, lungs and circulation.
- Third eye – an increase in psychic abilities and a stronger connection to the universe. This can be enlightening or even scary if you are new to this level of spiritual and universal connection. Physical symptoms that accompany this period are dizziness, hormonal imbalances, visual and hearing shifts, and balance issues.

It is recommended that during the 21-day Reiki cleanse, you should 'set the frequency at source', which is basically to focus on one symbol or Kotodama for three days, take a break, then use another symbol or Kotodama for three days and then take another break. This allows you to get to feel, know and understand the different frequencies, and the longer a person resonates at one frequency, the deeper the healing. But you should really trust your instincts and go with what feels right to you.

My experience of Okuden was very different from my Shoden cleansing. I was still in the mindset of 'the universe will make all my decisions', and before I returned from the Middle East a friend had asked if I would housesit for her whilst she tried to find a buyer for her home and I thought, *Why not?* So I was now back in London, waiting for a tax rebate from Mr Taxman, and basically spent six months reading my favourite books and getting lost in a world of fantasy. Sometimes solitude really is just another form of running away. Though my Shoden cleansing had been very positive, it was emotionally draining at times, so I felt lucky to have then found myself in a little house surrounded by books and in no hurry to get a job. Bliss, really.

I now did my Okuden with Tiffany and again my mind was blown. I remember thinking, *Wow, I now have the symbols and a cosmic bridge, and this healing energy is so much deeper.* I felt a deeper connection to the universe and a little high, yet grounded. I was going on another universal rollercoaster ride and this time it involved my heart on a much, much deeper level.

My friend sold her house and I somehow got my bank details wrong for Mr Taxman and was told I had to wait another six weeks for a cheque. So I packed all my belongings into storage and headed off to stay with my family for a few weeks.

A week into the visit, my maternal grandmother went into hospital with terminal cancer. To this day it has been the most heart-wrenching, heartbreaking thing I have ever experienced and I still feel the raw emotions now. It still feels so unfair that the universe would make such a beautiful, loving human being suffer so much. I had no job to go to or even a place to live, so it seemed right that I should spend this time with my family.

Having taken the Okuden a month before I moved to my family home, I had the tools and was able to send my grandmother 'distance Reiki' and also give myself Reiki to help deal with the emotional rollercoaster ride her illness brought. At the time, I was unsure if it was working for her, if it gave her any sense of peace, plus I hadn't asked permission so I felt a little guilty about it. Though I know she wouldn't have minded.

A couple of months later she passed over and I felt relief that she wasn't suffering any more, that she was free from pain. I remember feeling extremely exhausted by the whole experience. It's strange because, looking back, the whole experience is blurred, as if I walked through water the entire time, but the emotions are still raw, and very real. I was truly lucky in that I actually was there with my family and not running back to London or elsewhere for work. I got to experience something so personal with my family and for once not over the phone.

Reincarnation is part and parcel of many Eastern cultures, and having been brought up around these belief systems makes me more accepting of death. It is to me a part of the soul's life cycle, but the death of a loved one is always hard on the heart, regardless.

My Okuden cleansing happened at a time in my life when I was surrounded by loved ones whilst experiencing the harsh reality of cancer killing someone we deeply loved. Having the new symbols and giving myself self-treatments on a regular basis enabled me to share the loss with my family. Having the tools to heal on a deeper emotional level allowed me to come to terms with the death of my grandmother, but, heart of hearts, I still cannot accept what she suffered.

If I had not made that mistake on my tax return, I would have missed out on such a personal family experience, and so 'Thank you, Mr Taxman' for making me wait ages for my money. The universe does work in mysterious ways.

Overview of Okuden Symbols and Kotodama

Usui first used the Kotodama to teach his students how to connect to the different energy frequencies, and these have not been changed or adapted at all. The symbols are tools that Usui developed and introduced to some of his students who were unable to use the Kotodama. These symbols are rooted in Tibetan Buddhism and Sanskrit from the Indian subcontinent.

So what exactly are the symbols and Kotodama used for? Basically, once attuned and taught the symbols and Kotodama, you will be able to connect with different energy frequencies of the universal energy. These are used to heal different elements of dis-ease on a much deeper level. Hidden trauma and hidden dis-ease are very hard to detect, and it is human nature to ignore or avoid reaching into the deepest parts of our soul to confront these traumas and dis-ease.

Okuden gives you the ability to really cleanse on a deeper level. You will be able to feel the difference in the energy frequencies and use them to pinpoint different areas that need healing, for example emotional, mental or physical issues. You will also be able to send your Reiki healing to anyone, anywhere, to your past, your future and your relationships. The possibilities are vast.

Usui taught that these symbols and Kotodama are sacred and should not be shared with anyone who was not attuned at this level of Reiki. Originally the symbols and Kotodama were learned by meditation or committed to memory from teacher to student. Nothing was written. However, these symbols can be found inscribed on many temples and other buildings around Japan and the East, and so are not actually secret in the East. When Reiki was introduced to the West, manuals came into existence, and now via the internet the symbols and Kotodama are literally available to anyone who searches for them.

Today there are many different branches of Reiki, and that has resulted in different versions of the symbols being drawn and within Western Usui Reiki new symbols have been introduced. I personally think that it's not the actual symbols that are important but the intention with which we use them.

For many years I have questioned why the symbols and Kotodama should still be 'kept secret' from people who have not trained at this level of Reiki, especially as the information is so widely available and easy to find. Diane Stein first published the symbols in her book *Essential Reiki*, and for me that book was (and still is) an absolute must once I became a Reiki Master and when I first started teaching Reiki.

I feel that there needs to be a breaking down of barriers for more people to come into their own healing, for the highest good of the collective, of all of us on Earth. Being more open will allow people to learn more without the fear of commitment, let them explore what is for their own highest good. The world and information sharing has changed and it is time for Reiki to evolve again and become more inclusive.

However, even though the symbols and Kotodama are now so readily available, it doesn't mean that the symbols or Kotodama should not be sacred to you. When using the symbols or Kotodama, always give the highest respect. As a rule, if we Reiki Practitioners draw the symbols for ourselves, when they are no longer needed we burn them instead of ripping them apart. Burning them is more respectful, allowing the energy to transform and be released back into the universe.

Everyone is different and some people find it easier to connect to the different energy frequencies via the symbols and some via the Kotodama. Intention is key in connecting to the different universal energy frequencies, and Usui had intended that when a Reiki Practitioner was experienced enough, they would no longer require the symbols or Kotodama to connect to the different energy frequencies, as the intention itself becomes second nature and so the connection to the different energy frequencies becomes natural.

I must state, if you have taken the Shoden Degree, or are new to Reiki, be aware that you cannot just try to connect and give Reiki using these energy frequencies unless you have been attuned and connected directly to them by a Reiki Master.

We will explore the original symbols and Kotodama developed by Usui; however, I do recommend that you explore and discover different symbols that are used in different Reiki branches or any other energy healing paths, as you may connect more personally with different symbols and universal frequencies.

Cho Ku Rei – the Power Symbol

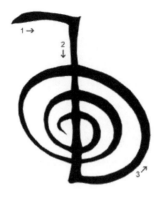

Public name: Power
Sacred name: Cho Ku Rei

Pronounced as 'show ko ray', this is the universal power symbol and commands that the power of the universe be here now. In Japanese Shinto magic, this symbol is used to turn wishes into reality.

In Reiki, this symbol relates to the Vajra in Tibetan Buddhism which was originally taken from *Vajra* in Sanskrit, which translates as both 'thunderbolt/irresistible force' and 'diamond/indestructibility'. In Hinduism the thunderbolt is held by the Hindu god Indra, and it can also be seen held by the Greek god Zeus and the Roman god Jupiter; even the Christian god has been depicted with a thunderbolt.

In Tibetan Buddhism, the Vajrayana school of Buddhism contains rituals said to allow a follower to achieve enlightenment in a single lifetime, in a thunderbolt flash of indestructible clarity. The Vajra is used as a symbol of wisdom, having power over illusions and evil spirits, which also accounts for Cho Ku Rei's abilities in cleansing and protection.

When researching the Japanese translation of Cho Ku Rei, I discovered that *Cho* actually has two different meanings, one of which is 'butterfly', but I was taught that the symbol's literal meaning translates to:

CHO – a curved sickle or sword that draws a curved line

KU – to enter and produce wholeness

REI – essence, universal power

Cho Ku Rei produces the densest energy frequency of Reiki and is geared towards the physical realm. Usui's surviving students described the frequency as earth energy, earth *ki*, the energy of physical existence. When using this symbol, it is always important to dedicate the energy for the highest good. If the highest good is different from what you wish for, it will remain working for the highest good regardless of what you want or think you need. When Cho Ku Rei is drawn and used in a treatment, the effect is twofold and the amount of Reiki being channelled is strengthened.

Following are a few examples of how to use Cho Ku Rei.

Physical healing:

Cho Ku Rei is a powerful tool for physical healing, in particular when focusing or intending that Reiki heal cuts, burns and so on. Cho Ku Rei only needs to be activated at the beginning of a treatment, but it can be repeated if you feel the need or if you are moving to another area of the body. Use your intuition and trust that Cho Ku Rei is working for the highest good.

Cho Ku Rei can also be activated to mend electrical objects such as lights and computers. I have heard of Reiki Practitioners using it to start up electric cars when their cars wouldn't start.

Space clearing:

Cho Ku Rei is excellent for clearing negative energies and can be used to clear your treatment room before and after a treatment, as well as your home, yourself, your food, clothes, crystals and such like. You can do this by activating the symbol and tracing it over whatever it is you wish to cleanse. In the case of a house or a room, you can trace the symbol over the walls, ceilings or floors or wherever you feel it is needed.

Protection:

The strongest form of protection is a positive thought, word or deed, but it is so much more powerful when activating Cho Ku Rei. You can activate the symbol over yourself, your belongings or your mode of transport.

Sei He Ki – the Harmony Symbol

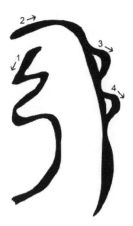

Public name: The Harmony Symbol
Sacred name: Sei He Ki

Pronounced 'see he key', this is the mental/emotional symbol and is the essence of compassion. This symbol allows one to transcend to a higher state of consciousness necessary to obtain enlightenment. Sei He Ki is said to bring about a mental spring-clean, to start afresh, and its literal meaning is as follows:

SEI – state of embryo, complete potential, which at the start is invisible

HE – relates to the root chakra

KI – energy

Sei He Ki generates a higher-frequency energy than Cho Ku Rei, and the energy frequency itself feels much lighter and delicate than the denser frequency of Cho Ku Rei. Sei He Ki is used to balance the emotional and mental planes. Usui's surviving students described it as the celestial energy, an energy that makes a link with the spiritual realm, and balances and harmonises.

The effect of Sei He Ki may seem less noticeable as it resonates at a much higher frequency, but it is just as strong as Cho Ku Rei. The energy can feel like a tickle, and sometimes it gives an instant emotional release, resulting in tears or giggles. However, most of the time the effects are subtle but strong.

When Sei He Ki is activated, the effect is again twofold. The amount of Reiki you are channelling is increased and the healing is geared to the mental and emotional bodies.

Mental and emotional healing:

Use Sei He Ki to deal with stress, tension, anxiety, insomnia, restlessness, trauma, anger, hurt, sorrow, grief and depression. In traditional Chinese medicine, various emotions are seen as being held in certain parts of the body; for example, anger is held in the liver, fear is held in the kidneys, grief is held in the lungs, joy in the heart, and sympathy in the spleen. So you can activate Sei He Ki in these body parts to release the blocked energies.

Positive affirmations:
Sei He Ki can be used for helping positive affirmation work; just slide your hands under the back of the head and repeat the affirmation to yourself whilst channelling Sei He Ki. Alternatively, after activating Sei He Ki, visualise the symbol moving into the brain, carrying the affirmation, and say the affirmation three times.

Relationships:
Sei He Ki is a very beneficial energy to channel when there is a lot of hurt. It is the energy of compassion, and drawing it over a room or bed, or channelling it through yourself when in the presence of someone who's hurting, is very empowering. As long as we let go of the outcome and dedicate it to the highest good, it can have some really beneficial effects.

Spirit rescue:
Sei He Ki can help spirit move over to the light, particularly if used in conjunction with the Connection Symbol. This is because both symbols are not physical, so they both resonate at the same vibration.

Activation of Cho Ku Rei and Sei He Ki
When using symbols, it is best to keep Cho Ku Rei and Sei He Ki apart. The symbols can be used on the same treatment; however, as the energies are different, it is best to activate them separately and on different parts of the body.

One Japanese school of Reiki states that Cho Ku Rei only needs to be activated once at the beginning of the treatment as it's so powerful. There is no need to activate it again during a treatment. However, you should use your own intuition and go with how you feel.

I was taught that when activating the symbols, you should say their names to yourself three times with each 'tap'. In Japanese Reiki, this is not done as it is considered that there is no need to state the obvious – use your intention. However, do say it to yourself if you find that it helps you focus on the symbol, and always dedicate it for the highest good.

To activate the symbols, do the following:

- Always visualise the symbol being drawn in the colour violet as this is the colour associated with Reiki, or if using on a certain chakra, visualise the colour associated with that chakra.
- Always 'tap' the symbol three times to activate its energy – visually or with your fingers or thumbs. You can draw the symbol on the palm of your dominant hand (onto the minor chakra in your palm) and then press both palms together three times to activate the symbol. Or you can draw the symbol onto your palm and activate it by tapping into your palm with your thumb three times.
- You can focus the symbols into a laser by drawing them with your thumb or fingers; this is useful for issues like toothache.
- You can visualise the symbol above your crown chakra and intend that it floods through your crown and out through your hands or even radiates out of every pore of your being, covering your client in a sea of Reiki.
- To change a symbol on your palm or the body, just rub or blow through the symbol. Or if visualising, see the symbol disintegrate before visualising the next symbol.
- I personally find that visualising the symbols and activating them whilst doing Reiji Ho is best for me. I visualise the symbols in my palms whilst my hands are in Gassho and tap three times. I then visualise the symbol

flooding the client's crown when I begin the treatment. I then use symbols as and when required, using my intuition.

Hon Sha Ze Sho Nen – the Connection Symbol

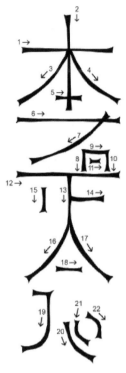

Public name: The Connection Symbol
Sacred name: Hon Sha Ze Sho Nen

Pronounced just as it is written, this is the symbol used to make a connection through the ethereal realm, to another time, place or person. It can be seen to mean 'The Buddha in me connects to the Buddha in you', and represents the Buddha consciousness, the ability of enlightened beings to extend their minds through time and space. Buddha consciousness includes all things, is infinite, and identifies with nothing. People who

74

have been initiated into this symbol and consistently practise it can experience progression of consciousness and increasing possibilities for transforming the ego.

The literal meaning is as follows:

HON – the centre, the essence, the source, the beginning, the start

SHA – shining

ZE – to walk in the right direction

SHO – the goal, the aim, honest being

NEN – silence, to be in the deepest core of your being

According to Usui's surviving students, this is the state of oneness. In the case of the Practitioner, it produces oneness with the universe, where distance or time does not exist. Take note that:

- Hon Sha Ze Sho Nen is not an energy that produces a particular frequency, as are Cho Ku Rei and Sei He Ki.
- It is used in conjunction with the energy frequency you wish to channel, for instance Cho Ku Rei or Sei He Ki.
- It may help you to see Hon Sha Ze Sho Nen as a cosmic bridge, something that is built to connect.
- Using Hon Sha Ze Sho Nen without a symbol would be like building a bridge that nothing ever goes across.

Connect to a person:

You can connect with a person with whom there is a physical distance, an emotional distance or a time distance by using Hon Sha Ze Sho Nen to build a bridge between you. Make a space for yourself that is peaceful and envision the person you wish to send Reiki to. Draw Hon Sha Ze Sho Nen and then the symbol/ Kotodama you wish to send, and envision it travelling over the cosmic bridge to the recipient.

Connect through time:

You can use Hon Sha Ze Sho Nen to connect with yourself in the future or past. The focus should be on ourselves and the situation at hand; for instance, you can send Reiki to yourself as a child during a traumatic time or to connect with your inner child. You will not be moving back in time; the healing takes place in the present, healing the effect it had on you.

Or for your future self, if you know an important date is coming such as childbirth, an exam, an interview or surgery, you can send Reiki to yourself to that time in the future, intending that you will be flooded with Reiki when you arrive.

You can also send Reiki to another person in your past or future, intending that they will be flooded with Reiki at the time required.

To send Reiki over time and space, visualise where and when you are trying to reach, activate Hon Sha Ze Sho Nen, and send the symbol/energy frequency you have chosen to cross over.

Connect chakras:

Hon Sha Ze Sho Nen can be used to connect any chakras you feel may need to work in more harmony with each other. For example, if you feel a more heartfelt communication is needed, draw a bridge between the heart and throat. Or if you need more creativity to come into manifestation, draw the bridge between the sacral and root.

Heal the world:

Hon Sha Ze Sho Nen can be used to send Reiki to world disasters such as tsunamis, hurricanes, floods, droughts, wars, and to Mother Earth in general. Just intend or see where you want the energy to go, draw the bridge and send it across.

Kotodama

The Kotodama are ancient, and the actual word translates into 'word spirit' or 'the soul of language'. Kotodama come from Japanese Shintoism, which is the indigenous belief system of Japan. In Shintoism it is believed that at the birth of the physical and spiritual world there was a Kotodama Suu and this developed into U, which then split into two opposing forces, A and O. In some respects it is similar to Om, which in Hinduism is the first sound/vibration that created the universe.

The Kotodama represent forces of the universe and there are a collection of 75 Kotodama which turn up in many aspects of Japanese life. They appear within Shinto and Buddhism as mantras for meditation, within martial arts and also in Reiki. There are historical accounts of Kotodama being used to stop armies, to heal, to kill and to control the weather. There have been accounts that state that the correct name for Kotodama is 'Jumon', which has connotations with magic.

There are probably less than a handful of Kotodama Masters left in the whole of Japan now. They take us back to the earliest of Japanese spiritual traditions, when it was believed that words had mystical powers and that saying something would make it so. Each syllable or Kotodama was thought of as a divine aspect of creation.

Some of the 'new belief systems' in Japan from the Meiji era to the present day have diagrams that show how each sound in the Japanese language creates and sustains the universe. The founder of Aikido Omoto-Kyo inspired Kotodama, and the 'Doka' poetry of Ueshiba was used in a similar way to how Usui used Waka poetry, as teaching tools with Kotodama contained within them, and it seems that Usui used other Waka poems, chosen because they contained Kotodama.

The Kotodama were the means by which Usui taught his students to connect with the different energy frequencies of Reiki. They predate the use of the symbols, which were introduced later as visual tools for Usui's students, who could not grasp the Kotodama. It is said that Usui worked with

77

his senior student, Eguchi, to develop the symbols with the intention that in time the students would no longer need the symbols and would work directly with the energy frequencies they represented.

Some people – and I am one of them – work better with visual aids than sounds or mantras. So you should use what you're comfortable with, as connecting with the energy frequency is the important thing, not how you connect.

The Kotodama are based on these basic vowel sounds:

A as in aaah
O as in rose
U as in true
E as in grey
I as in eeeee

Following are the pronunciations for the three Kotodama, Cho Ku Rei, Sei He Ki and Hon Sha Ze Sho Nen.

Name	Energy	Sound	Pronunciation
Power	Cho Ku Rei	ho ku ei	hoe koo ey-eeee
Harmony	Sei He Ki	ei ei ki	ey-eeee ey-eeee keee
Connection	Hon Sha Ze Sho Nen	ho a ze ho ne	hoe aaah zay hoe neigh

Kotodama meditations

To become more familiar with the energy frequencies of the Kotodama, chant them out loud. Sit comfortably with your hands in your lap, palms up, and close your eyes. Chant one Kotodama again and again with each out-breath. For the best effect, Kotodama should be chanted using a deep, resonant tone. Breathe them out of your entire body, resonate them from your dantien point, and sit quietly for a while and gently notice what impressions you get of the energies.

How to use the Kotodama in treatments

Either instead of, or as well as, drawing or visualising a Reiki symbol as you carry out a treatment, intone silently one of the Kotodama either three times or endlessly like a mantra. You do not need to say them out loud when you treat someone. The Kotodama should be used one at a time and not combined, the same as we would use the symbols.

Distance Healing

Distance healing not only works but is also very powerful. When working with distance healing, you are working without actual form but more in line with energies of the cosmos, and this is an integral part of Reiki.

In practice, when using Reiki for distance healing, it is normally only done for 15 minutes at a time, over a course of days. Some Practitioners will send it over 3–5 days in a row, at the same time each day. This is just a guide; you should always listen to your intuition. It is important to remember that it is the intention that creates the bridge for the healing, regardless of the methods that you use.

Below are some basic methods used for distance healing:

- Make an altar just for distance healing, which will allow you to focus your intention on building the bridge for the healing. Invoke the intended Kotodama or draw Hon Sha Ze Sho Nen and your intended symbol (Cho Ku Rei or Sei He Ki) over your altar and send the healing.
- Invoke the intended Kotodama or draw Hon Sha Ze Sho Nen and your chosen symbol over a teddy, doll or pillow and send Reiki to it with the intention that it is the recipient (person or situation).
- Invoke the intended Kotodama or draw Hon Sha Ze Sho Nen and your chosen symbol over your upper leg and send Reiki to your leg with the intention that it is your

recipient.

- Visualise holding the recipient in the palms of your hands as if you are holding a small ball safely in the palms. Invoke the intended Kotodama or draw Hon Sha Ze Sho Nen and your chosen symbols onto your palms and send Reiki to the space in your palms.

- Build up your connection to the recipient, and through your memories of them, try to visualise where they are. Invoke the intended Kotodama or draw Hon Sha Ze Sho Nen as the bridge and then your chosen symbol and send Reiki to them.

- Imagine a closed door and invoke the intended Kotodama or draw Hon Sha Ze Sho Nen over it and visualise the door opening and your chosen symbol being sent to the recipient with Reiki via the open door.

- Visualise a cosmic bubble which holds the recipient and invoke the intended Kotodama or draw Hon Sha Ze Sho Nen over the bubble and your chosen symbol. Imagine the cosmic bubble being flooded with Reiki.

This is very useful for people who can't be touched, for example a person with skin conditions, burns or new tattoos. It can also be used as a bridge to go to a certain area of the body like a major organ.

Ethics of distance healing

In Shoden we are taught that we do not give Reiki to someone without their permission. So it has been questioned whether it's ethical to send Reiki via distance healing to someone without their permission. It is always best to gain permission, but when sending healing to a situation, a past trauma, or an upsetting relationship, it is not always possible to gain permission.

The ethics of distance healing can be controversial and some people believe that if someone has not consented to the healing and you give it anyway, then that is a violation of that person's rights. This is something you need to be comfortable with. There is also the thought that if a person does not want Reiki, regardless of whether it's hands-on or distance healing, they will not receive it.

In some respects I think it may also be the same as sending prayers out to people. When sending prayers to people who have suffered or are suffering the hardship of war or a disaster, you are literally sending them love and healing via the cosmos. You don't contact them beforehand and ask them if they want your prayers. So why does sending out distance healing require permission?

I've had various experiences with distance healing, and in one case, two people were involved but only one was receptive to the healing. A client was suffering from bullying, which was really quite nasty and ego driven from a sibling. He was hurt, angry, and felt that he was in a really dark place because of things said to him by his sibling. The sibling was someone who blankly would have refused Reiki as it didn't sit well with his religious beliefs. However, he felt that as a religious person he had every right to push his views onto my client, who wouldn't conform to his brother's views.

So when sending the healing, I visualised them both as their younger selves, back in time when they had a lot of love and respect for one another. I put the two younger selves in a cosmic bubble and sent love. I asked the universe to help them remember that same love and respect they used to have for one another and to bring it back to them as they are now. I used Sei He Ki for this healing. I actually felt a resistance from the sibling. It was very strange. I could feel the love they had as their younger selves, but for some reason there was a real resistance from the sibling. Even his higher self was rejecting Reiki. So I decided that the best thing was to continue with the distance healing over a few days and focus all the intention on healing my client so his brother's negativity would not hurt him.

From this example you can see how distance healing may not work without someone's permission. Every single healing will be different, as is every situation and person involved. Whatever does happen, it is good to remember that if someone wants Reiki, they will receive it. If they don't, well, they won't.

However, if you really don't know whether to send distance healing, try this little exercise. When thinking of the person, switch Reiki on but do not direct it at them. Just focus on the energy and let it heal the part of you that wants to send it. Reiki should always be about the self, first and foremost, so heal the part of you that is stuck in the situation.

Energy Meditation Exercises

When we spend time 'becoming or being at one' with the different energy frequencies of Reiki, we can connect to them on a much deeper level. The most effective way to do this is to meditate on the symbols daily by first looking at them, then spend time with your eyes closed, visualising them and seeing them in your mind's eye. Or with the Kotodama, chanting them over and over in a meditation.

The following exercises were in the Okuden Manual that I received and I have found these to be useful, so have included them. The exercises should help you to 'feel' the different energies. As stated before, Cho Ku Rei is a much denser energy and so you should be able to feel its vibration. Sei He Ki is softer, but again you should be able to sense its vibration.

Energy exercise 1:

1. Sit comfortably with your eyes closed and your hands on your lap, palms facing upwards.
2. Visualise Cho Ku Rei in the air above you being 'tapped' each time you say its mantra – three times.

3. Imagine cascades of energy flooding down on you from the symbol, through the crown and hands, flooding through your entire body.
4. Try the above with Sei He Ki, and though you won't feel an energy as such with Hon Sha Ze Sho Nen, try to sense the bridge.

Energy exercise 2:

1. Sit comfortably with your eyes closed and your hands in your lap, palms facing upwards.
2. Visualise Cho Ku Rei up in the air above you being 'tapped' each time you say the mantra.
3. As you breathe in, draw the energy down through your crown, hara line and into your dantien.
4. As you pause before exhaling, feel the energy build.
5. As you exhale, flood the energy through your body out into your aura.
6. Try the above with Sei He Ki, and though you won't feel an energy as such with Hon Sha Ze Sho Nen, try to sense the bridge.

Energy exercise 3:

With a partner, channel the energy of Cho Ku Rei and Sei He Ki through to them. Then find out if they could feel the energies. People normally describe Cho Ku Rei as thick, dense, solid, heavy and coarse, or treacle-like. People normally describe Sei He Ki as being fine, delicate or ticklish, and wispy.

Japanese Techniques and Treatments for Okuden Level

Usui was known to use many different techniques in Reiki treatments, which continued to be used in Japan by his surviving students. It was when Frank Arjava Petter went to Japan and found some of Usui's surviving students that a lot of Usui's original techniques were discovered, and he then introduced these techniques to Western Reiki. The following techniques were taught by Usui to students doing the Okuden Degree.

Koki-Ho – healing with the breath method

If you feel hot during a Reiki treatment, it is an indication that you are full of Reiki energy and your hands can't administer it fast enough. In cases like this, it is useful to use either Koki-Ho or the next technique, Gyoshi-Ho.

1. Inhale, drawing your breath down into your Tanden (the energy centre located deep inside the hara, roughly midway between the top of the pubic bone and the navel).
2. Hold there for a few moments whilst you draw Cho Ku Rei on the roof of your mouth.
3. Exhale and breathe the symbol over the area to be treated or into the aura. It is helpful to visualise the symbol at the same time.

Gyoshi-Ho – healing with the eyes method

Gyoshi translates as 'staring', but here we are using a soft focus, not an actual hard stare. You have to relax and soften your focus to be able to 'look' through an energy field.

1. Soften your focus and look through or past the physical, into the energy field of that which you are treating.
2. Allow the energy to travel into your third eye, making an energy circuit between you and the recipient.
3. You can then project the symbols you wish to use with your eyes.

Tanden Chiryo – Tanden treatment

Tanden Chiryo is used as a general power-up technique for yourself or others. It is also used to strengthen willpower.

1. Place one hand on your Tanden and the other on your back, level with the Tanden.
2. Keep both your hands in place until they lift off by themselves.
3. To power it up further, use Cho Ku Rei.

Gedoku-Ho – detoxification method

Ge means 'to bring down' and *doku* translates as 'toxin'. This technique is used to help reduce any detoxification and is also useful for reducing the side effects of medicines.

1. Place one hand on the Tanden and the other on the back, level with the Tanden.
2. Visualise all the toxins running out from the body down into the earth where they transform into nourishment.
3. It will help when treating someone if they join in the visualisation.

Reiki Undo – Reiki exercise

Undo translates as 'exercise'. This exercise is literally about undoing the restrictions found in the body and is a useful exercise to do.

1. Give yourself an area with enough space to move around freely.
2. Start in Gassho, asking for Reiki Undo to commence.
3. With your arms fully outstretched, make fists in both hands with your thumbs enclosed.
4. Inhale deeply through your nose.
5. Exhale vigorously through the mouth whilst pulling

your arms tightly into yourself and tighten all your muscles.

6. When all the air has escaped your lungs and your arms are tucked back with your fists near your shoulders, let go completely, allowing your arms to fall where they wish to fall.

7. Allow your lungs to fill with air on their own.

8. Repeat three to five times.

9. Inhale deeply and let go as much as you can, then exhale. Repeat, breathing deeply until your body wants to naturally move. Be patient; if your body is not ready to move, keep breathing until your body is ready.

10. Then let your body move, however it wants to move. Let it flow. Resist the temptation to make your body move or to stop it from moving. Just flow.

11. If you are finding it difficult to move, give yourself permission to be as free as a child for the next 20 minutes. Allow yourself free rein to laugh, cry, yawn, let go of any wind, or scream if that is what your body wants to do. Just don't think. Allow your body to flow and do what it needs to do.

Ketsueki Kokan Ho (Kekko) – the massage procedure

Kekko is a massage that is used at the end of a treatment, and the exact sequence with photos can be found in the *Hayashi Reiki Manual*, page 55. The wording may be a little different from the original, though, due to translation. This is a delicate massage and not one that requires you to be a massage therapist or have any massage experience – though I would suggest practice makes perfect. This is a massage that is beneficial to regulate blood pressure.

I was first taught a shorter version of Kekko during my Okuden 2nd Degree, but when researching a Japanese Reiki school called 'Jikiden Reiki', I discovered this procedure.

Tadao Yamaguchi, who set up the school with his mother, Chiyoko, wrote a book called *Light on the Origins of Reiki*. This is a wonderful story of how Reiki did survive in Japan and was used and taught in a family environment before they set up the school. It also gives a great insight into how Reiki is taught and viewed in Japan, along with basic guidelines and so on. I recommend reading this book. Chiyoko was taught Reiki by Dr Hayashi as a teenager.

The Kekko massage sequence follows. Before starting this massage, ensure that your client is lying face down and wearing light clothing.

1.   Find the indentations located on both sides of the neck at the base of the skull. Place your thumb and index finger there and draw with your fingers Cho Ku Rei to intensify Reiki energy in both sides, once each. By doing this, Reiki goes to the head. Locate the spine.

2.   Place your index finger and middle finger on either side of the receiver's spine. Quickly slide your fingers down along the spine (from the bottom of the neck to the sacrum). Repeat 20 times.

3.   Find the indentations on the sacrum. As you did in the neck area, place the thumb and index finger there and again draw Cho Ku Rei on either side, once each. This sends Reiki through both the upper and lower body of the receiver. Divide the upper part of the body into five or six areas. First place your palms on the upper area on either side of the spine, and then slide your hands down to the sides of the body. Do the same on the remaining parts. Repeat this three or four times.

4.   Rub across the small of the back, sliding your hand from side to side (back and forth) with slight pressure. Repeat ten times.

5.   Outsides of the legs: Start from the hip area and brush

your hand down along the outside of the leg as far as the ankle. Repeat this three or four times. Do the same on the other leg.

6. Backs of the legs: Start from the back of the thigh. Again brush your hand down from the bottom of the buttocks to the ankle. Repeat this three or four times. Do the same on the other leg.

7. Insides of the legs: Separate the legs a little. Start from inside the thigh and brush your hand down as far the ankle. Repeat this three or four times. Do the same on the other leg.

8. Pushing down on the base of the thigh with your left hand, clasp the ankle with your right hand. Using your body weight, stretch the back of the knee. Repeat the same on the other leg.

9. Pat all over the back of the shoulders down the rib cage to the lower back and to the buttocks. Repeat this three or four times.

10. Pat down the legs in the same order as in 5, 6 and 7. Start from the outside of the leg, then the back and finally the inside of the leg. Right leg and left leg alternately.

Genetsu-Ho – technique for bringing down a fever

Ge translates as 'bring down' and *netsu* translates as 'fever'. This is a technique that Usui used to treat any disease of the head:

- Give Reiki to the forehead, temples, back of the head, neck, throat, crown, stomach and intestines.

Hesso Chiryo – the navel healing technique

Hesso translates into 'navel' and *Chiryo* translates as 'treatment'. This technique is used for re-energising and rebalancing. You can use this on yourself or others; however, ensure that when treating others they don't mind being touched in a sensitive area such as the belly button. Also ensure that your touch is very gentle.

1. Place your middle finger in the navel and apply a slight pressure until you feel a subtle pulse. You are not trying to detect the pulse of the abdominal aorta deep in the belly. Instead try to sense the energetic pulse that can be felt by touching the belly very gently.
2. After locating the pulse, let Reiki flow out of your middle finger until you feel the pulse and energy in harmony.

Professional Reiki Practice

As stated, professional practice of Reiki is only allowed once the Okuden 2nd Degree Reiki Course has been completed. So following is some information regarding how Reiki is regulated in the UK.

The body that represents Reiki Professionals in the UK is the Reiki Council. The Reiki Council has affiliated with the General Regulatory Council for Complementary Therapies (GRCCT), which means they are the federal regulating body for Reiki Practitioners. The framework for Voluntary Self-Regulation (VSR) is the National Occupational Standards (NOS). The NOS was developed to ensure that Reiki Professionals work within clearly defined professional standards. The NOS set the minimum standard required for professional Reiki practice. This allows for the dual effect of both protecting the general public from poorly trained Reiki Practitioners and driving up the standard of Reiki offered professionally.

Reiki Professionals can register for VSR by registering with GRCCT. However, this is not a legal requirement at present in the UK. I do advise that if you wish to practise professionally, you keep yourself updated on any changes to the regulations and UK law.

It is also advisable to get Reiki Insurance and look into

getting it tied in with Public Liability Insurance, which you will need if you are working from a home base or working at public events.

I should also state that currently it is the Reiki Practitioner/ Master who is regulated and not Reiki itself.

For useful information see the website of the UK Reiki Federation – www.reikifed.co.uk – for the latest regulations, legislation, general guidance, insurance and so on.

Professional Reiki Treatments

Following is guidance for when treating clients in a professional treatment.

Before they arrive:

1. Check your hygiene. Good practice equals fresh breath, clothes, clean hands and a good deodorant.
2. Make sure everything is ready – that the room is warm and there are extra blankets if required. Check that phones are switched off and you won't be disturbed.
3. If you have time, do a little meditation and send out your intention into the universe.
4. If you have time, recite the Five Principles and practise Hat Su Rei Ho or the other Japanese techniques used before a treatment.

When they arrive:

1. Client Information Forms – these are private and confidential and should not be shared with anyone without the client's permission. The forms should be filled in before a treatment and should include the following questions for the client:

    a. Do they have a pacemaker? There is a theory that

Reiki will interfere with pacemakers and so it is important to explain this to them. I was advised to not do a Reiki treatment on someone with a pacemaker; however, I have had clients with pacemakers and I just ask them to keep an eye on them.

b. Do they have diabetes? If they do, ask them to check their blood sugar levels before their next injection after the treatment as it can make a difference.

c. Are they pregnant? Reiki is great for unborn babies, but there have been cases of women having miscarriages and then threatening to sue the Reiki Practitioners. (I have not heard of any successful claims.) It is always best to inform the pregnant client and let them decide. But you also have to ensure you are comfortable practising Reiki on a pregnant woman.

d. Do they wear a hearing aid? Clients with hearing aids can experience pain so it is always best if they remove them for the treatment.

2. Ask the client to remove any jewellery, watches, belts and glasses. There is a theory that metal can interfere with a Reiki treatment by blocking the energy from going to all the places it needs to go to. However, I only ask clients to remove jewellery if they are wearing a lot and it will interfere with hand positions. I personally believe that as Reiki is the universal energy, it can penetrate through metal, but the general consensus is to remove it.

3. Play some soft meditation music in the background that allows the client to feel more comfortable. Sometimes clients may prefer sounds of nature like birdsong or waves, but general loud noise like traffic can be distracting for both the Practitioner and the client.

The treatment:

1. Ask the client to lie down on the massage table and get comfortable. I leave it to the individual clients to lie on their backs or fronts. If a client has a back problem, sometimes it's easier for them to have a pillow under their knees or to sit in a chair. It's important that the client is comfortable and in a pain-free position.

2. Explain that all they need to do is lie down and allow time for themselves. So long as they're comfortable and warm, they should feel relaxed. Many clients fall asleep.

3. Sit or stand by their head, put your hands in Gassho, and ask Usui or the universe for permission to be a channel for the highest good of 'your client's name' (say this aloud or in your mind). At this point you can also ask if any angels, guides, ancestors and so on would like to join in with the healing.

4. Scan the energy around your client to see if any symbols or Kotodama come to mind and then activate the one that you're drawn to.

5. Place your hands around the head but not touching it, then scan with your hands to find any Byosen. Ask your client if they are comfortable with you actually touching their head, as the heat coming off your hands can be uncomfortable for the client. If the heat or touch is uncomfortable, keep your hands at least 2 or 3 inches away.

6. When you move your hands above the eyes or the throat, do keep your hands a few inches above the skin.

7. Remember to keep a dignified distance from intimate areas.

8. It is not necessary to move a client from lying on their back to lying on their front, as Reiki will go wherever it is needed. However, if a client has back problems the

heat from your hands may be nice on their back.

9. If you feel any tingling or a lot of heat from your hands in a certain area, this could be indicative of a 'Reiki hot spot' (a place that is very receptive to healing); just keep your hands there until it dies down.

10. If you find that during a treatment you feel emotional, start coughing, your belly rumbles or you feel any pain at all, remember that this is just temporary and that Reiki is clearing negativity from the recipient. Whatever you feel will pass and you are always protected as Reiki passes through you too.

11. If you feel coldness over an area, this is usually indicative of a very old block. If you sense a magnetic pull towards it, keep your hands there, as it could be that it is ready for healing. If, however, you feel your hands being repelled from a certain area, go to the outer edges of the cold spot and place your hands on either side of it or above it by a few inches.

12. If you ever feel that the client is blocking the Reiki (most likely on a subconscious level), then they are probably not ready for the healing. Just keep going until the treatment has ended.

13. During an emotional release, a client may start crying or laughing uncontrollably. If this happens, just put your hands on their shoulders until they have calmed down. Then continue with the treatment.

14. If a client wants to stop the treatment, stop. Sometimes it can be uncomfortable for them. Never take this personally – remember detachment.

Finishing the treatment:

1. After spending a good amount of time on the feet, come up to the head and smooth down the aura by lifting up

your hands as high as possible and slowly bounce them down until you feel a resistance (the client's aura/energy field). Then brush down along the aura, from the head to their feet three times, with the intention of clearing away any negativity and settling down their aura. Then disconnect by blowing through your hands.

2. Put your hands in Gassho and thank Usui and the universe for the Reiki.

3. Place your hands on the client's shoulders and ask them to sit up when they are ready.

4. Wash your hands with cold water as this helps to clear the Reiki energy at the end of the treatment. I usually leave the room to wash my hands and give the client a little time to come back into themselves.

5. Offer them a glass of water.

6. Ask them how they feel. They may wish to discuss the experience or ask you if you felt anything. Try to keep anything you say in a positive manner. Never diagnose.

7. Explain that they may experience a cleansing period for a few days and advise them to drink lots of water to assist the cleansing.

8. Make sure they are grounded before they leave.

Grounding:

After a Reiki treatment the Practitioner and/or client may not feel grounded, which is basically a state of feeling light-headed and slightly unstable on their feet. Food, especially root vegetables, help to ground, as well as drinking water.

If you or your client are both not feeling grounded, lie down on the floor or sit down, close your eyes and breathe deeply, filling your lungs. Imagine roots coming out of you, breaking through the floor, breaking through the layers of the ground below and anchoring you straight to Earth's core. Continue breathing deeply and feel gravity weighting you down.

General Guidance for Reiki Practitioners

Most people who take Okuden do not actually want to be professional Reiki Practitioners, and they are happy with self-treatments and only giving Reiki to family and friends. But if you do feel that you want to practise Reiki professionally, I would generally recommend that you allow time for the cleansing period. Give yourself at least six months because your cleansing is working on a much deeper level and, unlike Shoden, it is harder to define, and to feel.

Okuden opens you up to your deeper self and this brings with it many lessons. One of the things my Reiki Teacher taught me was 'Love, the higher kind, is all you need', and this lesson has stuck with me ever since. Always remember the old saying, 'Healer, heal thyself', and also that to give Reiki, which is love, we need to give ourselves love first. If you have doubts or concerns, look to Reiki to find your path. Try to stay in line with your intuition and your integrity, and if you experience negativity, allow it to open you up and take a look at why you react or feel the way you do.

Following are a few pointers to remember for new Reiki Practitioners:

1. Unless you are a doctor or medical professional, never diagnose. It's against the law.
2. Client Information Forms. It is important to note that these forms are private and confidential and should be treated as such. Without a client's written permission to share their information, you could be in breach of data protection laws.
3. We never force Reiki on anyone and we don't do Reiki on anyone we're uncomfortable with.
4. You are not responsible for the client's healing. They are.
5. You are just a channel for Reiki. There needs to be detachment from the outcome.

6. You are in a very honoured position and you must remain worthy of that – respecting each individual and practising a non-judgemental attitude, keeping confidentiality, staying neutral yet compassionate, with empathy, not sympathy.

7. Some people don't like to be touched, so always check with them first and then just keep your hands a few inches off the body. Never touch a person's genitals or breasts.

8. Always work from the head to the feet, spending ample time on the head and feet and smoothing down the aura at the end.

9. If ever working on a child, I would also ask the child if they want Reiki, just in case it's being pushed onto them and to ensure that they are comfortable and that they want it.

10. You should never do Reiki on broken or cracked bones until a medical professional has reset them properly first, as Reiki can result in the bones healing before they are in the position they should be. Always get the bones reset and then apply Reiki to quicken the healing process.

11. If you ever feel aroused during a Reiki treatment, do not worry about it. It rarely happens and being aroused is a normal part of being human. Send the aroused feelings down through your feet to ground them. It could be that the client has issues in this area and you are just picking up on them. Do not be alarmed and do not overthink it. Just release it.

12. Always 'ground' your client at the end of a treatment, to bring them back into themselves.

Chapter 3

Shinpeden and Shihan Master Degree of Original Usui Reiki

Eastern and Western Philosophies

Introduction

On the Shinpeden and Shihan Master Degree we explore further symbols and Kotodama, the Attunement process, the Reiju Empowerment process, and how to teach Reiki. This is the final Reiki Degree but the beginning of your Reiki healing and learning on your soul/spirit/deepest energy level.

On the Shoden 1st Degree, the energy channelled when initiated is Cho Ku Rei, which is geared to cleanse and heal the physical – your physical body and physical environment. On the Okuden 2nd Degree, the energy channelled when initiated is Sei He Ki and together with Hon Sha Ze Sho Nen is geared to cleansing and healing the mental and emotional and deepening your connection to the universe. On the Master Degree, the energy channelled when initiated is Dai Ko Myo, which is geared to cleanse and heal the spirit. It is easy to overlook the possibility that the soul/energy body may be carrying the burden of dis-ease and so many people can neglect this level of healing.

Usui only initiated around 20 people to Master level as he believed that spiritual development could take a lifetime. He developed a structure for his Reiki courses in a way that practised mindfulness, discipline and spiritual growth, and by following his teachings and incorporating them into our lives, we are able to connect so much deeper with the universe. The Master initiation allows us to really see who we are on a spirit level and how we are connected to the universe, enabling us to fully embrace our highest potential.

The Master Cleansing

As with every Degree, once attuned we embark on a 21-day self-treatment, and as a student on this Degree, the focus is on cleansing the spirit, which can uncover deep blocks and trauma that we are unaware of consciously. We should be in a mental space where we enjoy the self-treatments, but I've found that the Master cleansing can be quite uncomfortable. It's also very hard to define and pinpoint what is healing and see the progress at the time. It's when we look back that we can see how the cleansing worked for us. On the other hand, some may swim quite easily through the Master cleansing; it really is unique to each of us.

The Reiki Master will join the students on a 21-day Reiki cleanse and, as a Reiki Master, it doesn't make it any easier. You never know what those shifts are going to release, and with each Attunement you give, you will receive one. So if you have three students on a one-day course, you could receive nine Attunements and three Reiju Empowerments and this can leave you feeling exhausted.

As all our chakras are spiritual, they will all go through the cleansing and shifting; however, the crown and third eye chakras are the spiritual chakras and the cleansing can or will have profound results.

Cleansing of the crown chakra can result in a period of general disorientation, doubting, questioning and searching for something but not knowing what. This cleansing can affect you mentally and emotionally. On a physical note, you may have ailments around the head and body. This period, however, may lead to an eventual general feeling of knowing your part in creation, and having faith and trust in yourself and the universe. You develop an understanding of your connection to the greater consciousness and an increased ability to channel spiritual energies or become aware of other vibrations.

Cleansing of the third eye chakra can result in feeling unbalanced, unclear and confused on the mental and emotional levels, as well as (or maybe followed by) possible physical ailments with hormones, eyes, nose, ears, sinuses and balance – leading to an eventual general feeling of more balance, clarity, intuition, empathy and increased psychic sensitivity.

Shoden guided me to *me*, in such a way that I could see myself, my past, my personal traumas, and learn how to honour and appreciate the lessons of my past and who I had become at that moment in my life. Okuden guided me to my heart, to my family, to experiencing my greatest loss whilst being in a place of love. The Master Degree, however, gave me a proper kick up the arse in the most gentle of ways, and in turn guided me to my soul. The healing allowed me to see that I needed to take back control and live again, to feel fulfilled again. To claim back my passion for life again.

After my maternal grandmother passed, my parents went abroad for a few months and I spent this time with my paternal grandmother. Now my paternal grandmother and I didn't really speak the same language, but we communicated well enough. She was old and not well, and she had all these little habits that I conformed to because they comforted her in a way. For example, my grandmother liked to go to bed at 9 p.m. and she pretty much bugged me to come upstairs too. I'm not sure, but I think it made her feel safe to know I was just a few metres away.

It was a very quiet time for me. In the morning my grandmother would be picked up to go to my aunt's house and come back late afternoon. We spent the evenings watching the TV with the volume so low (she didn't like noise) I could barely hear it. I cooked for her and basically looked after her. Having lost my maternal grandmother, I was grateful to have this time with my paternal grandmother, but I was still living in the mindset of 'the universe will make all my decisions' and I was walking in circles not achieving anything.

I had the opportunity to pop over to London and take my Master Degree with Tiffany, and having the Master symbol really took my Reiki healing to much deeper levels, levels I was unaware of. I connected with my paternal grandmother in a way I hadn't before. This may sound strange, but cleansing with the Master symbol opened my heart to my grandmother in such a way that I saw her in a completely different light. She became more than my paternal grandmother. She became a woman with a history, with a story to tell. She had a crazy sense of humour which I had never realised I shared with her. I saw myself in her and her in me. My grandmother was a healer on so many levels. I saw her. And so, I began to see myself.

My parents returned and my mum started to nag me about leaving home and going back to London to basically 'get a life'. I still didn't want to take back the responsibility of making all my decisions, and in many ways I was still as lost as I had felt before I took the Shoden Degree, but I was no longer angry or bitter. It's so easy to hide from living, from life. Yes, I had healed many parts of me, but I still felt lost. Then something occurred to me. I would always be lost, and only I could find myself. This in itself was a big wake-up call. The universe had taken me under her wings and it was time for me to learn to fly again.

A part of me didn't want to leave the safety of my parents' home, but I wasn't living, just going from one day to another. Yes, I had needed the time with my paternal grandmother, especially after losing my maternal grandmother in the way we did. But a great part of healing from trauma is learning to go out and start again. Live again. This can be so hard, to take that first step back into the world. I began to feel a need to see my friends, to start going out and socialising. I began to feel a need to connect with my old life in London, I began to miss the London life and I, yes I, made the decision and I moved back to London. I was lucky to stay with a friend until I found a job and a little flat in Brixton.

The main thing that the Master cleansing taught me was that I had a habit of letting others make my decisions so I didn't have to face the responsibility of being in charge of my own life. It was so easy for me to just give up on myself and let the universe guide me. Yes, I honoured my past, but I was in many ways still hiding from myself and I wasn't honouring who I was in the present, or my future self.

The Master cleansing allowed me to see and connect much deeper on my soul level. It allowed me to wake up – to see that I needed to live and only I could make that step. Instead of being a prisoner of my own fears, I began to crave a freedom only I could give myself, and once I had make the decision to reclaim by life, I began to feel at peace with myself and, most importantly, I began to live again.

Now that's my Reiki cleansing through the Degrees, but it's not the end of my healing journey. Reiki has become part and parcel of my life story, and my healing continues.

Overview of Master Symbols and Kotodama

There are four symbols and one Kotodama which are normally taught in Original Usui Reiki Master Degree, as below:

- Usui Dai Ko Myo – Traditional Eastern Master Symbol
- Tibetan Dai Ko Myo – Non-Traditional Western Master Symbol
- Tibetan Fire Snake
- Raku

Usui used the Usui Dai Ko Myo during his Reiju Empowerments to connect his students to Reiki. For Western Attunements, either Dai Ko Myo can be used, but it should be noted that the Tibetan Fire Snake and Raku are not essential and a lot of Reiki Masters do not use them.

What I do think is important is that the symbols or Kotodama are a means of recognising the different energy frequencies. After a while of using them, you should be able to connect with the different energy frequencies without relying on Kotodama or symbols. We become 'one' with the frequencies.

Reiki, as Usui taught it, was uncomplicated and simplistic. Getting caught up in complicated rituals takes away the focus of Reiki, so it is important to just let Reiki flow. It may feel hard at first, but practice makes it easier.

Usui Dai Ko Myo – Traditional Eastern Master Symbol

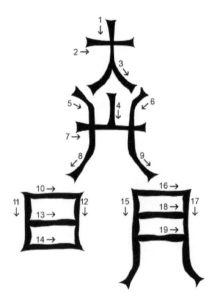

Public name: Master

Sacred name: Dai Ko Myo

Pronounced 'dye ko me-o', the Usui Dai Ko Myo is made up of three kanji which translate as 'great bright light'. There are various definitions available, but one which was used by Hawayo Takata is, 'Praise be to the great universal light of transcendental wisdom'. It can also be read as to mean 'the universal life force coming together with spirit'.

The Usui Dai Ko Myo symbol is the most powerful of the Reiki symbols, which is why it is called the Master symbol. It is believed that Dai Ko Myo combines the power of Cho Ku Rei, Sei He Ki and Hon Sha Ze Sho Nen and is the heart of Reiki. Dai Ko Myo connects the spirit directly to Reiki.

This is a very old symbol that has been used in Japan for centuries and can be seen in many Buddhist temples. This symbol was used for manifestation work and was deemed so powerful that it is said it was used to manifest the results of war, as well as everyday wishes such as inner peace, success and healing, not just for people but also for situations. So, as a rule in the East, it has never been a secret symbol as such; however, it should still be sacred to you.

The Usui Dai Ko Myo was represented as 'the key to the light', the 'key to the system', a representation of the ability to transfer the Reiki ability to another. A symbol that allowed you to fully connect with the soul. Ultimately, this symbol is about being at one with the universe, our soul merging with the universal energy. This cannot happen with a simple Reiju Empowerment or Attunement. It comes with the realisation that we are 'one'. You are the universal light and the universal light is you.

The Usui Dai Ko Myo symbol represents empowerment, intuition, creativity and spiritual connection. It enables recognition and clarity about your true path in life. Dai Ko Myo activates a powerful energy for self-empowerment and is used for opening spiritual connection, intuition and healing on cellular and genetic levels.

Usui Dai Ko Myo allows us to fully connect with our soul body and heal trauma or dis-ease which is carried deep in our souls. This is the soul cleanser, the soul medicine, the soul healer. It is this 'oneness' with the universal life force that allows blocks in our soul to be cleansed. Now not everyone has the same beliefs, but if you are open to it, Dai Ko Myo can heal trauma and disease from past lives, future lives, parallel lives, by connecting our soul with Reiki. Regardless of our belief systems, everyone who uses Dai Ko Myo has the ability to heal the spiritual/deeper energy body, which can then have a knock-on effect and heal the physical body, mind and heart.

Dai Ko Myo when used regularly will improve your intuition and psychic abilities. When meditating with Dai Ko Myo it can bring enlightenment and peace and can change your entire outlook on life. This symbol brings you into your own power, into your spiritual power, and is perfect for manifestation work.

In Western Reiki Attunements, the Dai Ko Myo symbol is used and seen as essential for passing on Reiki to the recipient by connecting the recipient's soul to Reiki. Some Reiki Masters will use the Usui Dai Ko Myo whilst others will use the Tibetan Dai Ko Myo. However, I must stress that it doesn't matter which Dai Ko Myo symbol you use. As always, it is the intention and focus that is important.

When you get to first feel both Dai Ko Myo, you may find that there is a difference in the way both energy frequencies feel. Usui Dai Ko Myo has a lighter feel to the energy frequency than Tibetan Dai Ko Myo. It is said that Usui Dai Ko Myo is a deeper cleanser than the Tibetan Dai Ko Myo, so for a more gentle soul-cleanse, some Reiki Masters prefer to use the Tibetan Dai Ko Myo.

Tibetan Dai Ko Myo – Non-Traditional Western Master Symbol

The Tibetan Dai Ko Myo, or Dumo as it is also known, is not a traditional Reiki symbol or a traditional Tibetan symbol. It was introduced into Western Reiki by an American man called Arthur Robertson who was the only Master student of Iris

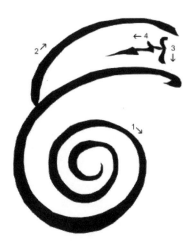

Tibetan Dai Ko Myo

Ishikuru (one of Takata's students).

It is thought that the actual symbol has its origins in Hindu philosophies and represents the swirling fiery heat which ascends up and over the spine as a result of *kundalini* awakening – the unification of mind and body working with the fire in the base chakra.

Some Reiki Masters state that the energy frequency is slightly denser than Usui Dai Ko Myo. Its energy is likened to a spiritual Cho Ku Rei. Its primary use is that of a cleanser, and this is used to pull out negative energy or dis-ease from a body, a room or a situation, and release it. Therefore some Reiki Masters during a Reiki treatment will use Tibetan Dai Ko Myo to clear any blockages before using the Usui Dai Ko Myo to enhance the healing.

However, I must state, so as not to cause any confusion, that in a Western Attunement you can use either Usui or Tibetan Dai Ko Myo. In a spiritual healing, again, you can use either symbol. They both connect to the frequencies that unblock, cleanse and heal the soul.

Tibetan Fire Snake

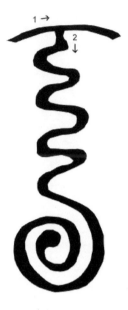

Tibetan Fire Snake

The Tibetan Fire Snake is another symbol which is believed to have been introduced into Western Reiki by Arthur Robertson and is not considered to be Tibetan in origin. It originates from the Hindu philosophies of kundalini, and the snake-like coil represents the kundalini energy in the base chakra as it rises up through the chakras, opening them up.

Many Western Reiki branches use the Tibetan Fire Snake at the beginning of Attunements to open, cleanse and join up the chakras, bringing them back into equilibrium, ensuring that the chakras are open for energy to flow through the recipient during the Attunement.

The Tibetan Fire Snake can also be used for a Reiki treatment and is drawn over the recipient's body at the start of or during a treatment. Again it opens, cleanses and joins the chakras, aiding healing and clearing away negativity.

Raku

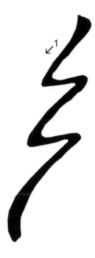

Raku

Again, Raku is not a traditional symbol that is used in Japanese Reiki. The symbol is considered to be Tibetan in origin and is used by Buddhists to enhance enlightenment by drawing it up towards the sky.

Raku is associated with Western Reiki and is used at the end of an Attunement by the Reiki Master, who will draw it downwards to ground the recipient, seal in the symbols and Reiki itself to the recipient, and then disconnect the energy from the Master. Again, like the Tibetan Fire Snake, it is not used by all branches of Western Reiki and not all Reiki Masters will use it.

Raku can also be used at the end of a Reiki treatment to ground and disconnect from the recipient if drawn downwards.

Kotodama

Following on from the information on Kotodama in the Okuden manual, below is the Kotodama for Usui Dai Ko Myo.

The basic vowel sounds are:

A as in aaah
O as in rose
U as in true
E as in grey
I as in eeeee

Below are the pronunciations for the four Kotodama, Cho Ku Rei, Sei He Ki, Hon Sha Ze Sho Nen and Usui Dai Ko Myo.

Name	Energy	Sound	Pronunciation
Power	Cho Ku Rei	ho ku ei	hoe koo ey-eeee
Harmony	Sei He Ki	ei ei ki	ey-eeee ey-eeee keee
Connection	Hon Sha Ze Sho Nen	ho a ze ho ne	hoe aaah zay hoe neigh
Master	Dai Ko Myo	a i ko yo	aaah eee coe yo

Overview of Reiju Empowerments and Attunements

At each level of the Reiki Degrees, the Reiki Master acts like a channel to initiate a student to a particular level of Reiki by giving them an Attunement or Reiju Empowerment. This means that the Master passes on the ability to connect to the Reiki frequencies. Attunements and Reiju Empowerments serve the same purpose, though there are a few differences.

Reiju Empowerment is a Zen-like energy practice that Usui developed and used to pass on the Reiki ability to a student and can be used also to empower yourself with Reiki. This was only used in Japan by Usui's students until it was spread to the West in the 1990s. Some believe that Reiju Empowerments continue to work, rather than the instant blast of Attunements.

Attunements were developed by Hayashi and taught by Takata as a heavily detailed ritual used to pass on the Reiki ability to another. This was the sole method of passing on the Reiki ability in the West until the Reiju Empowerments were discovered.

During Attunements and Reiju Empowerments some people have profound experiences, whilst others may feel nothing at all. These affect everyone differently as our vibratory rates are different and are instantly raised by being connected to Reiki. That which is vibrating at a lower level (trauma, negativity), and no longer serves you, will be released during the cleansing period.

The Hui Yin Point and the Violet Breath

The Violet Breath is in some Reiki paths considered to be of much importance when conducting the Attunement process; however, it is not vital and a lot of Reiki Masters don't do it. Again, it is the intention of passing Reiki on to another that is the most important element of an Attunement.

Oriental medicine works on the basis that there are a set of 12 pairs of meridians (energy points) running along the length of the body and two meridians channelling energy along the front and back of the body in the mid line – the Functional and Governor Channels.

The Hui Yin is considered to be an important energy gateway, and by contracting the Hui Yin Point, you are keeping the life energy in the body and raising it to the higher energy centres. When giving yourself or someone else a Reiki treatment or an Attunement, by connecting to this energy gateway, you can maximise the benefit of Reiki entering your body.

To connect to this energy gateway:

1. Contract your Hui Yin Point (located in the perineum, which is a pressure point felt as a small hollow between the anus and the genitals).
2. Press your tongue on the roof of your mouth.
3. The Hui Yin Point is contracted by pulling your pelvic floor gently into the body, holding it and then gently releasing it.

This is a gentle pull and you should not be pulling any other part of your body.

To start, try 20 quick in-and-out releases, then hold it for 20 seconds. Contracting the Hui Yin Point does take a little practice, but soon you will find that it comes naturally.

The Violet Breath is your breath when contracting your Hui Yin Point. You breathe it out when breathing out from your Hui Yin Point.

It should be noted that Usui did not use this during his Empowerments and (as far as I'm aware) it is not used in any Japanese Reiki.

The Attunement Process

The Attunement works by the Reiki Master opening up the crown chakra and passing the Reiki energy through the upper chakras and out through the minor chakras in the palms of the hands.

I recommend practising the ritual until you are confident of the moves before initiating a student. It should feel natural as if you're flowing through the movements. I started off practising on a pillow placed on a chair until I was able to flow with the movements, but I kept my notes close the first time I gave an Attunement and, luckily enough, practice ensured I didn't have to look at them.

Before starting the Attunements, get yourself in a relaxed mental and spiritual state. I normally give myself a Reiju Self-Empowerment and meditate before the recipient arrives. Ensure that the room is warm and quiet and that you will not be disturbed.

To start, the recipient should be sitting comfortably on a chair with their back straight (use a cushion if required) so their chakras are in line and their feet are firmly on the ground. Make sure that you leave enough space around each recipient for yourself to move around. Ask the recipient to close their eyes and put their hands in Gassho and meditate on receiving the universal energy.

Normally for Shoden 1st Degree, three Attunements are given; however, some Reiki Masters will repeat Attunement 3, so four Attunements are given in total. Other Reiki Masters give three Attunements and also include a Reiju Empowerment.

I've put the following symbols down as this:

Dai Ko Myo – DKM
Hon Sha Ze Sho Nen – HSZSN
Sei He Ki – SHK
Cho Ku Rei – CKR

I've included in the Attunement rituals a detailed longer version and also a short and simple version. This is so you can see what the basic Attunement is like and, as stated before, not everyone uses the Tibetan Fire Snake, Raku or the Violet Breath. Practise and see what comes to you naturally.

Shoden Attunement 1:

1. Invite the recipient to sit on a chair with a straight back. Ask that they close their eyes, be quiet, meditate on receiving the universal energy and put their hands in Gassho.
2. Stand behind the recipient, put your hands in Gassho, and ask Usui and guides to be present for the Shoden Attunement 1 and for guidance.
3. Draw DKM (Usui or Tibetan) onto your palm and press three times into the other palm to transfer the energy.
4. Draw Reiki symbols DKM, HSZSN, SHK and CKR into the room to fill it with Reiki.
5. Connect and hold the Hui Yin position, with your tongue at the roof of your mouth, throughout the Attunement.

Hold your breath unless you are blowing and then hold it again.

6. Open the crown of the recipient by drawing the Tibetan Fire Snake from their crown to their root with the intention of opening up their energy field.

7. Step into their energy field and place your hands on their shoulders; close your eyes.

8. Build up your Violet Breath.

9. Place your hands on the recipient's crown and visualise the crown chakra opening as you open your hands and blow the DKM symbol into their crown. See the symbol moving to the base of their brain. Visually tap the DKM symbol three times.

10. Raise the recipient's hands above their head (still in Gassho) and draw CKR in the air above their hands. Visualise the symbol moving into their hands and crown as you visually tap the symbol three times.

11. Move the recipient's hands back to their chest and move round to their front. Open their hands out flat, holding one of your hands underneath to support them.

12. Draw CKR in front of their third eye, tapping towards it three times.

13. Draw CKR in front of their hands three times, visualise CKR moving into their hands, and press your thumb three times into their palms.

14. Place the recipient's hands back into Gassho and let go.

15. Blow the energy from their hands down to their root, up to their crown, back to the root and up to their hands with the intention of flooding their hara line.

16. Move behind the recipient and place your hands on their shoulders for a few moments. See a ball of light entering their crown and moving to their heart, carrying a positive affirmation: You are a channel for Reiki for evermore.

17. Place your thumbs at the base of their skull and say to yourself, 'I seal this process with divine love and wisdom.' Visualise a door with CKR being closed. Say to yourself that the process is now complete.
18. Place your hands on the recipient's shoulders and visualise brilliant white light bathing you both.
19. Move back, Gassho, bow and then draw Raku from crown to root of the recipient with the intention of disconnecting and grounding the energy.
20. Disconnect and release from the Hui Yin position.
21. Thank Usui and guides and take a break.

Shoden Attunement 2:

The exact same steps as in Shoden Attunement 1, but in step 10, raise the recipient's hands above their head (still in Gassho) and draw SHK and CKR in the air above their hands. Visualise the symbols moving into their hands and crown as you visually tap the symbols three times.

Shoden Attunement 3:

The exact same steps as in Shoden Attunement 1, but in step 10, raise the recipient's hands above their head (still in Gassho) and draw HSZSN, SHK and CKR in the air above their hands. Visualise the symbols moving into their hands and crown as you visually tap the symbols three times.

Shoden Attunement 4 is not required, but if you want to, repeat Shoden Attunement 3.

Short and simple Shoden Attunement 1:

1. Invite the recipient to sit on a chair with a straight back. Ask that they close their eyes, be quiet, meditate on receiving the universal energy and put their hands in

Gassho.

2. Stand behind the recipient, put your hands in Gassho, and ask Usui and guides to be present and for guidance.

3. Visualise the recipient's crown chakra opening and blow the DKM symbol into their crown. See the symbol moving to the base of their brain. Visually tap the DKM symbol three times.

4. Raise the recipient's hands above their head (still in Gassho) and draw CKR in the air above their hands. Visualise the symbols moving into their hands and crown as you visually tap the symbol three times.

5. Move the recipient's hands back to their chest and move round to their front. Open their hands out flat, holding one of your hands underneath to support them.

6. Draw CKR in front of their third eye, tapping towards it three times.

7. Draw CKR over their palms and press your thumb three times into their palms.

8. Place the recipient's hands back into Gassho and let go.

9. Blow the energy from their hands down to the root, up to the crown, back to the root and up to their hands with the intention of flooding their hara line.

10. Move behind the recipient with the intention of closing their aura, keeping the symbols inside. (Do not close the crown chakra.)

11. Move back, Gassho, bow and thank Usui and guides and take a break.

Okuden Attunements:

On Okuden only two Attunements are given, as follows:

- **Attunement 1.** The same process as Shoden Attunement 1, except in steps 10, 12 and 13, you draw and place HSZSN and SHK before drawing CKR.

- **Attunement 2.** Repeat of Attunement 1.

Shinpeden and Shihan Master Attunements:

On the Master Degree, only two Attunements are given, as follows:

- **Attunement 1.** The same process as Shoden Attunement 1, except in steps 9, 10, 12 and 13, you draw and place HSZSN, SHK, CKR and DKM.
- **Attunement 2.** Repeat of Attunement 1.

The Attunements can use up a lot of energy for both the giver and receiver, so after the Attunements it is good to do some grounding, and have a drink and a snack of some kind.

Reiju Empowerments

The word *Reiju* can be translated in two ways using Japanese kanji, one way meaning 'accepting spirituality' and the other way meaning 'giving spirituality'. Spirituality in this case means the connection to Reiki energy.

Other translations that I've found are 'union of mind and *ki*', and 'the giving of the five blessings/powers', which refers to the five hand positions that are held after the crown has been opened during a Reiju Empowerment.

A Reiju Empowerment is considered to be much more than an Attunement in that it connects Reiki to the recipient and continues to reinforce the connection, increasing the strength of the recipient's Reiki and enhancing their spiritual development. The more someone receives Reiju Empowerments and works with the energy, the further they develop their intuition and sensitivity to Reiki energy.

Reiju Empowerments are what Usui developed, used and taught, and they are still used by the Usui Reiki Ryoho Gakkai. The information on Reiju Empowerments was first introduced to the West by Hiroshi Doi, who taught a version of Reiju taught by the Gakkai, and his technique is based on his experience of receiving them at the Gakkai.

The Reiju Empowerments included in this manual were passed on to Chris Marsh by one of Usui's surviving students, and are as I was taught and still use whenever I give an Empowerment.

Reiju Self-Empowerment

Reiju Self-Empowerments can be used to open up and connect to Reiki before giving a recipient a Reiju Empowerment or a treatment.

1. Raise your hands to connect with Reiki, palms facing towards the sky.
2. Feel Reiki cascading down into your palms, filling your hands, arms, torso and dantien point.
3. Bring your hands slowly out to the sides, palms facing the floor, intending that as you do so, you are bringing energy in through your crown.
4. Keep moving your hands down to the dantien point with the dominant hand hovering closer to your body and your non-dominant hand covering but not touching, flooding the energy over and through your body into your dantien point.
5. You have now surrounded yourself with the energy and brought it into your dantien point.
6. Hold this position until you feel a real sense of connectedness with Reiki.
7. Repeat the process three times.

Self-Empowerments can also be used to open and connect a group of students. Whilst doing the Self-Empowerment, you can expand the energy to engulf the group, thus connecting them also to the sacred space.

The Reiju Empowerment Process

Before starting the Reiju Empowerment, make sure that the room is warm and the recipient is sitting comfortably on a chair with their back straight (use a cushion if required) and their feet are firmly on the ground. Make sure that you leave enough space around each recipient for you to move. Ask the recipient to close their eyes and put their hands in Gassho and meditate on receiving the universal energy.

Following is the process to give Reiju Empowerments.

Reiju Empowerment:

1. Start with a Reiju Self-Empowerment.
2. Stand in front of the recipient, Gassho and bow.
3. Move your hands high up above you and feel Reiki energy coming into your hands from above.
4. Energy path: Move your hands down a little and join the first two joints of your index fingers with the others, floppy and relaxed.
5. In one continuous movement, move your hands down in front of the recipient and draw a line of light which enters the crown and trace an energy path down the centre of the body to the bottom of the spine, intending that you are opening up the energy centres as you go.
6. Part your hands and with your palms face down, move your hands sideways past your knees and down to the floor, ritually grounding the energy without coming into contact with the floor. Move your hands to the sides as you stand up.
7. Now you are going to be holding a number of hand positions where you will be flooding an area with energy. Each position should be held for at least 10

seconds, but at the same time try to treat it as a graceful, flowing dance.

8. Crown: Stand up and move to the side of the recipient. Move your hands down so they hover at the point of the aura surrounding the recipient's crown, your non-dominant hand over your dominant hand, palms down but not touching. Open the crown (visualisation and intention) and direct the energy down the energy path you traced.

9. Temples: Standing in front, follow the outline of the aura and slide hands to both sides of the temples. Visualisation and intention should be focused on directing the energy to flood the whole body with Reiki.

10. Third eye: Following the outline of the aura, move your hands to the front of the recipient's face and make a triangle with your thumbs and index fingers. This is said to be the symbol of the sun. Hold the centre of the triangle in front of the recipient's third eye, intending that you are flooding it with energy. This is said to help the third eye function more sensitively and connect with higher consciousness.

11. Heart: Stand to the side of the recipient. Hold your hands in front and behind the heart centre and flood it with energy.

12. Hands: Touching the tips of your first three fingers, move your hands down around the recipient's hands, cupping your hands around them but not touching. Flood the hands with Reiki.

13. Finishing: Move your hands up over the recipient's fingers and bring your hands smoothly down towards their knees (fingertips still touching). Smoothly separate your hands and, with palms facing downwards, move your hands sideways past their knees and down towards the floor, starting to scoop round in a circle.

14. With the intention that you are scooping up excess energy and returning it to the source of the Reiki, bring your hands together just above the floor (making contact with your two little fingers as if you are scooping water from a stream). Quickly move your hands up, pointing your fingers towards the centre of the recipient's body as if you are scooping up the energy and returning it to the sky, returning the energy along the pathway you first traced. As your hands reach towards the sky, open your arms, releasing your little fingers.

15. Gassho and bow.

It is a good idea to take a 15-minute break after each Reiju Empowerment to allow the recipient to just breathe, and for yourself too. There is a lot of energy being used, so many people feel cold after being initiated or in need of a snack or hot drink.

Reiju Empowerments and Kotodama

Following is what was passed on to me regarding the number of Reiju Empowerments conducted on each Degree and the responding Kotodama to use, if required. Kotodama are not essential for Reiju Empowerments, but if used, they should be intoned when visualising and flooding the crown, temples, third eye, heart and hands with Reiki energy.

- Shoden 1st Degree – one Reiju Empowerment is given but no Kotodama.
- Okuden 2nd Degree – three Reiju Empowerments are given in total and the Kotodama used are:
  ∘ 1st Reiju Empowerment – Cho Ku Rei
  ∘ 2nd Reiju Empowerment – Sei He Ki
  ∘ 3rd Reiju Empowerment – Hon Sha Ze Sho Nen
- Master Degree – one Reiju Empowerment is given using the Kotodama Dai Ko Myo.

Distance Attunements and Reiju Empowerments

As with distance healing, distance Attunements and Reiju Empowerments work just as strongly as one-to-one sessions. When conducting a distance initiation, it is a good idea to speak to the recipient, see a photograph of what they look like, and know exactly where they will be. This helps with the intention and focus when conducting the initiation.

Set up your space as if conducting a one-to-one Reiju Empowerment and imagine that the recipient is sitting on your chair but wherever it is that they are, and conduct the initiation as if they are on that chair. Visualise Reiki entering them and connecting them. Practice helps to smooth out the movements and visualisation.

Teaching Reiki

As your cleansing will take six months or longer, I do recommend taking this time to focus on your cleansing and healing and, if interested, maybe practise teaching and passing on Attunements and Reiju Empowerments. Some Reiki Masters don't teach and there is no reason for you to feel that you should, but when and if you feel you would like to teach Reiki, the following may be of guidance. Start by teaching Shoden first, and when you are comfortable, take on Okuden students and then the Master students.

The universe will send to you students for your own highest good, and to your students you are the teacher selected for their highest good. The longer you teach, the more confident you should get, but always be aware that you may get students who challenge what you think you already know. I've found that I've learned a lot from my students, mostly about myself.

Following are a few pointers and things to be aware of, but always follow your instincts and make your courses your own.

Timing

Plan ahead and decide if your courses are to last one day or two days and how much content you want to go over and discuss with your students. Ensure that you time the course in advance, including the Attunements, Empowerments, and any breaks you will have. Keep to the time. Initiating others to Reiki will use up a lot of energy so you need to consider how the energy also affects your students and try not to do too much in one day.

Structure of courses

I structure my courses around the content in my manuals, spacing the different topics and exercises with breaks and time for the Attunements and Empowerments. I find this keeps the course as simple as possible and allows me to keep an eye on the time and not rush.

Typically I structure a one-day Shoden course as follows:

10:00   Start: Introduction and overview of Reiki
10:30   1st Attunement
11:00   Overview of the cleansing period
        Exercise: How to feel your own aura
11:30   Overview of Western philosophies
        Western hand positions and self-treatment exercise
12:30   2nd Attunement
12:45   Lunch
13:15   Overview of Japanese philosophies
14:00   3rd Attunement
14:30   Overview of treating others
15:00   Exercise: Giving Reiki to another and receiving Reiki
16:00   Reiju Empowerment
16:30   Other treatments and any questions
17:30   Finish and relax

It looks like a lot to get through in one day so I normally only do one-day courses for one or two students. I do ensure that all the students are given a manual at the beginning of the day so they can make notes as required and are able to refer to them when required. I also ensure that they are aware that I am available for any support or questions after the course. After their 21-day Reiki cleanse, I contact them to get any feedback.

Some Reiki Masters may only give an overview of Reiki and a manual of the hand positions; it depends on their Reiki path. The emphasis, I think, should be on connecting the students to Reiki, giving them the basics and then setting them off on their healing path. As always, Reiki is your students' teacher as Reiki is your teacher.

Practise in advance

Practise, practise and practise how to pass on Reiki to another. The more you know the structure of the Attunements and Empowerments, the easier it flows and the easier it is to just focus on the intention of passing on Reiki.

I also recommend practising teaching the course before giving your first course. I did this before my first course, mostly because I wanted to ensure I had the timing right but also because I was nervous and wanted to get it all right. I wanted to sound like I knew what I was talking about, and it did really help in making the first day run smoothly.

Number of students

My first course had only one student and it took place over two days as I wanted to go over all the information in as much detail as possible. I think the student left feeling overwhelmed. It was a big learning curve in keeping the courses simple and remembering always that this isn't about me as a teacher, but it's about a student taking a big step in their own healing and learning.

I now prefer to have two students over one day and give

them all the basic information, plus time to ask questions, and also give them time to practise on themselves and each other. They have all the details in the manuals so have something to refer back to if need be, but I also encourage them to research and explore all the different paths for themselves. As per my first course, I discovered that if you give them too much to think about, it can take away from the experience and confuse them.

My Reiki Teacher used to have up to eight students over two days, but she also had someone assisting her to pass on Reiki. What worked for her does not work for me. I find too many students can really drain my energy levels, so I stick with what I am comfortable with. It is good to remember that you too are receiving an Attunement, and this energy shift really can have an effect on you and deplete your energy levels.

Pricing of course

Depending on where you live and work, the price you can charge for a Reiki course can differ. I took all my Reiki Degrees at a well-known establishment in London with an experienced Reiki Master. So I expected the costs to be much higher than in other parts of the UK. However, that does not take away or add to the value or quality of the Reiki courses I took or actually teach.

Before I started teaching, I researched what the other local Reiki Masters were charging for their courses and I also looked at their content, how long their courses are, and how well established they are. I keep my prices in line with the local competition, though once a year I do promote discounted courses for one month only.

We can always give discounts, but attempting to undercut the competition – other Reiki Masters – and trying to steal students with lower than average prices goes against what Usui taught. It takes the love and healing out of Reiki and seems to be more about ego or fear of not earning enough. But we must also never undervalue Reiki, for what it is and all the lessons it teaches us.

Layout of manuals

You will find that most Reiki manuals are similar in that they contain the same information, and many even have the same layout. This is because of the way Original Usui Reiki is structured: within each path of Reiki, the information is the same.

I based the structure of my manuals on the manuals I was given by my Reiki Teacher but rewrote them from my personal angle, still passing on the basic principles, exercises and meditations. Over time I've added and taken away contents, but I've always kept all the basic teachings and information in place.

I do recommend getting your manuals and other teaching tools in place before you start teaching Reiki. Get to know your manuals inside out and all the information within them, adding your personal experiences and how they are relatable to Reiki in general.

Things that should be included in manuals depend on what path of Reiki you are teaching, but the basics are as follows.

Shoden:

- The history and development of Reiki
- The different elements of Western philosophies, including chakras and hand positions
- The different elements of Japanese philosophies, including the Japanese meditations, energy exercises and the Five Principles of Reiki
- Self-treatments
- Basic information on how to treat others
- Ethics, detachment, the responsibility of healing, and so on

Okuden:

- The symbols and Kotodama
- Distance healing
- How to treat others in a professional environment

Master:

- The symbols and Kotodama
- The procedure for Attunements and Reiju Empowerments
- How to teach others

General Guidance for Reiki Master

As Reiki Masters, we are in a place of responsibility, and that involves not only teaching the basics of Reiki but also ensuring we have given our students the tools to go out and follow their own path, wherever that leads them.

We must always remember to be detached. Do not get attached to your students' learning; they are on their own journey. We pass on Reiki to them with all the basic information and then step back. Though we share a part of each other's Reiki journeys, we still walk them alone in our unique path.

We do not force people to take courses and I never book the next course straight after one has been taken. I encourage the student to take six months to focus on their cleansing and then only contact me if and when they are ready to take the next Degree. They may take it with another Reiki Master, they may decide to take a different healing path, or they may end their courses there. That is their path and their choice.

It is true that the Master Degree takes you on a spiritual journey that really is not expected. It's hard to see the cleansing, the healing, until much later when you have more understanding of who you are on a deeper spiritual level. The connection to the universe via the Master initiation is beyond what I thought I knew, and it has grounded me and given me a foundation which I never knew I had. A spiritual foundation which supports me on this path, helping me adapt and grow and find my highest potential at any particular moment in time.

Chapter 4

After the Reiki Degrees

You will find that most of your Reiki learning will take place after you have finished the Reiki Degrees. The cleansing and healing can, over time, change the way you think, the way you feel, and the way you react to situations and people. You may find that you become passionate about things you never gave a thought to before, and you really don't care about things you were once passionate about. It's a journey of self-discovery which takes time to explore and then one day you realise that you have really found your place in healing, and you have made it your own. You become the healer your soul always knew you were. For many Reiki Masters, Reiki is more than healing; it's a tool which enabled them to find who they really are, and become their highest potential.

I personally think it's really important to find your own path in healing. There are many different paths and it really is important to find a place where you are comfortable, and to do the things that are natural to you, even if others may not agree. Some Reiki paths, I find, are rigid and have so many rules that I found them to be constraining instead of liberating. Healing should feel free of restrictions and the healing energies should flow naturally, and this can take time to achieve.

My learning certainly continued after I finished my Reiki Degrees, and it still continues. I am still learning and growing and becoming more and more comfortable with who I am as a healer. I learn, I adapt the learning to suit me, and I continue to learn and adapt. We should never put ourselves in a place where we believe we have learned all there is to learn, because that is the one thing that will stop us from growing as healers. There is always so much more to learn.

Additional Symbols I Use

Reiki is adaptable and we as Practitioners should be able to adapt with Reiki and with whatever life brings to us. There are many who stick to certain 'rules' in Reiki, and that is fine if it is what serves them best, but as individuals in a world that requires so much healing and cleansing, we must recognise that we are unique, our healing is unique, our path is unique and it is OK for our Reiki practice to be unique as well.

Do not be afraid to adapt and change your healing practices, to learn from other paths, to grow and find completely different ways to connect to the universe.

What is the most important thing in connecting to Reiki is the intent and the intention of what we are doing. Without intent there is no healing or cleansing or connecting to the right frequencies.

There are so many different symbols available and they each have their own unique frequency and powerful vibration, some of which you may find that you really connect with and some that you don't connect with at all. There are Reiki Practitioners who adapt symbols or connect to different healing-energy frequencies to work for them in ways they probably wouldn't work for others. It is unique to us all and intention is always key.

Experiment and get to know the different frequencies, how they feel and heal, and adapt Reiki to suit you, your strengths and your knowledge.

I too have adapted Reiki to suit me and my needs, so it works better with my skills and knowledge and so I'm not spending so much time on thinking of rituals but just intending and doing.

The following two symbols are ones that I use on a regular basis side by side with the original Usui symbols.

The Spiral Funnel – My Cosmic Bridge

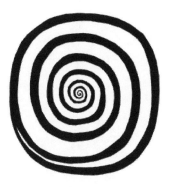

The Spiral Funnel

I've included the Spiral Funnel though it is not an actual symbol as such, but it is something that I actually use whenever I need to build a cosmic bridge. I believe that Reiki is unique to each and every one of us and, for some strange reason, I never found the same connection with Hon Sha Ze Sho Nen, and this symbol/ image would always pop up and Reiki would flow down the Spiral Funnel to wherever it needed to go.

Whenever I've given distance Reiki treatments and also when attuning a student using the Spiral Funnel as the cosmic bridge, I have never had any negative feedback or a lack of Reiki being sent to wherever it needs to go. I treat this symbol with the utmost respect and in just the same way that I respect Hon Sha Ze Sho Nen; I just resonate with the Spiral Funnel more. As always, and this is very important, it is the intention that matters.

Mer Ka Fa Ka Lish Ma – the Mother/Goddess Energy

This symbol represents the 'Mother/Goddess Energy' and is the DNA activator symbol. When used in a Reiki treatment it helps to restore/restructure DNA back to the original blueprint

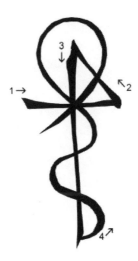

Mer Ka Fa Ka Lish Ma

or purest form before trauma or dis-ease became a part of us. Repeating Mer Ka Fa Ka Lish Ma as a mantra is soothing like a meditation and it just takes me away to a place of healing.

I was first introduced to this symbol when I first became premenopausal and was finding it difficult to balance all the hormonal changes that were occurring at the time. So I used this symbol and chanted the name on a 21-day Reiki cleanse and, with the help of supplements, my hot flushes calmed down, and my hormones began to rebalance. I was not only able to limit the extreme changes to my body, mind and hormones but also found that I was beginning to embrace the changes.

I feel pleased with myself for getting here, and I laugh at myself for my brain fog, though a few of the physical symptoms are really uncomfortable. But the fact is I made it to this point in my life and it gives me a freedom I never appreciated before. I'm free from having to dye my hair or my roots, because I like the colouring of my new-found white hairs. I feel proud of my body and how I look, and I tell my body that I love her and will take care of her. I have a freedom to cry whenever I want and about anything I want, because I see it as a five-minute release that allows me to breathe.

I also suffer from trigeminal neuralgia, which is basically damage to the facial muscles, ligaments and nerves from grinding my teeth my entire life and can cause extreme pain in the face and head. The first time I experienced the pain, it lasted for about 12 weeks non-stop and I was physically unable to do anything. The doctors gave me muscle relaxants but they just gave me a painful stomach. However, when I started a 21-day Reiki cleanse using Mer Ka Fa Ka Lish Ma, alongside facial massages and facial exercises, I was able to keep the extreme pain at bay.

I spent months waiting for a hospital appointment and if I hadn't done the facial exercises and Reiki, I wouldn't have been able to work because of the pain. When I did finally get a hospital appointment, I was lucky that the doctors advised acupuncture – provided on the National Health Service – to relax my facial muscles and an extremely rigid gum guard to stop the grinding and any further damage. I'm happy with this route as I prefer not to take medicines that just cause other problems, but I know that using Reiki with Mer Ka Fa Ka Lish Ma really did assist with relaxing my muscles to a point where I could at least get through the day without taking painkillers, though I do take some if I can't control the pain.

Mer Ka Fa Ka Lish Ma is a symbol I use and one that I find I really connect to.

Finding My Highest Potential with Reiki

After completing the Master Degree and moving back to London, I somehow thought that this would be it – that my life would fall into place and I would remain a Londoner living the London life. I worked as a site office manager for a developer/construction company which specialised in building luxury apartments, a project which was to last three and a half years, and I rented a lovely little flat in Brixton. I was surrounded by friends at work and in my private life. It was very much a 'work hard, play hard' kind of lifestyle. It was fun. I felt like I belonged and I did whilst I was there.

However, when I look back now – and I wasn't aware of this at the time – I see how slowly I actually began to change my outlook, my lifestyle and the direction of where my life would go. I began to seek a quieter life and spent more time in silence. I listened more to the nature that was around me. I was lucky enough to walk along a part of the River Thames every day on my way to and from work, and it was a quiet part of the river. Every day I listened to the river and tuned in to her life-giving and nurturing power.

At home, my little flat looked out on gardens full of birds singing and I was lucky to have quiet neighbours. However, the area was built up and I began to feel claustrophobic. A deeper part of me was yearning for open spaces. I have always been a big-city girl, but I've always loved the sea and wanted to move to the seaside. I found myself in a place where I was surrounded by friends, in a city I love, but I craved to be by the sea, or by a forest, to be in nature and not surrounded by concrete and brick.

In many ways, I found that I still needed guidance, that I still felt as if I didn't have the right direction in my life. Everything I thought I was, and everything I thought I needed, began to somehow feel wrong and trapped, but I didn't know what was right for me. I wasn't lost as such, mainly because I felt quite grounded and surrounded by love, but I felt that I had maybe outgrown the city lifestyle. I found I didn't want or need its noise any more.

I have found as I've got older, as I've grown as an individual, that my needs have changed, and what was no longer serving me had to change. I recognised that I needed more guidance, and instead of looking for the universe to take me under her wings again, I pushed for the change that needed to take place.

I booked myself on a six-month spiritual/life-coaching course which really looked at my fears, what caused them and how they were stopping me from finding my true potential. The course itself included life coaching, Reiki, tarot and lots of cleansing and healing. Each month I had to make myself do certain things that I felt uncomfortable doing, ticking them off on a list. Things like dancing by myself in public – sober, trying to talk to people I didn't want to talk to, reminding myself every morning on the Tube that all the people who were crushing me were tiny little cosmic souls in the same situation as me. I was put in situations where I was not confident or comfortable, but I knew I needed it and it was my Reiki cleansing that had put me in a place where I knew I had to break barriers that I had built over many lifetimes.

One of the things about this course which I found difficult at the time, even as a Reiki Master, was recognising all my flaws on a much deeper level – seeing my flaws not just in this life but also in my past lives and working out how trauma from past lives affected me now. It was, I suppose, a continuation of my Master cleansing, but one in which I was ready and so able to really see and admit to behaviours that I had subconsciously hidden before.

A part of the course was focused on me learning to trust myself completely to make my own decisions and see them through, and towards the end of the course I made a commitment to myself that I would practically and physically change my life for the better. I was afraid to love, to allow love into my life, and one of the things I had to push myself to do was join a dating site. I don't like dating sites and it was uncomfortable, but I committed to it, though I still had a few doubts.

I met my partner on the dating site – this 'perfect for me' man who I never thought could be real, and there he was living by the sea, available and interested in me. Reiki healing allowed me to break down barriers and open myself up to love, to whatever the future brings. I met him towards the end of the site project, so the timing seemed perfect. As my work came to a close, I moved to a pretty little seaside town to be with my new love and fulfil the dream of living by the sea.

I couldn't find work so I set up a Reiki business and I was lucky that my partner supported me in being free to find myself in this new situation. Transition was hard and at times uncomfortable, but it felt right, and over the past few years I've continued to grow, to evolve and to find myself on deeper and deeper levels. If I had stayed in the city, I would never have started my own Reiki business and I would have missed out on so much learning and developing.

I know this isn't my final stop. We both have a need to go more rural and plan to move again to a place where we have land to roam. Though we walk this path together now, we are both fulfilling our own unique and individual needs.

What I've found throughout my personal Reiki journey is how resourceful Reiki actually is. Whenever I have troubles, a physical issue or feel out of sorts, I turn to Reiki. Whenever I feel negative energy in a situation or a location or with a group of people, I turn to Reiki. Whenever I need lifting I cocoon myself in a Reiki bubble. I give myself 21-day Reiki cleanses whenever I feel a need to connect on a deeper level or if I'm dealing with pain or dis-ease. It's now in my psyche as the go-to resource. Reiki in many ways is my companion, my teacher and, to be fair, my reality checker or arse kicker.

However, and I cannot stress this enough, if I need to see a medical expert, I do, and I will take any medicine that the doctors see fit because they are the medical experts. Yes, I include Reiki in all or any healing that I need. I believe that Reiki will benefit any healing required, by clearing away any blocked energy, and that it works hand in hand with medicine to improve my health and well-being.

Reiki is, however, more than just a companion to any medicine I receive. Reiki has given me the tools to really accept myself and, alongside the Five Principles of Reiki, has taught me to evolve and grow whenever I've needed to. The Five Principles of Reiki have taught me that self-love and self-discipline go hand in hand together. Loving and taking care of myself is something that I still battle with, but it has also made me very aware of the fact that I alone am responsible for my actions, words, life. Without the tools of Reiki, I have no idea where I would be right now, but I do know that I would probably be living and working in toxic environments and still have toxic relationships. Reiki has allowed me to remove the dis-ease, the drama, and the behaviour patterns that kept me in trauma.

At each point of my life since I first learned Reiki, I have had to grow to be the person I needed to be at that particular point in my life. I've had to find my highest potential at that moment in time and it's not been an easy ride, but it's allowed me to see who I really am, flaws and all, and that has given me the tools to grow into what I needed to be.

Reiki has allowed me to slowly but surely remove all the layers that I thought the world had put on me to conform to. Reiki has allowed me to see that I only belong to me and I am responsible for me. I love my partner and family, but they don't belong to me and I don't belong to them. I and they are our own unique little cosmic beings with our own unique paths. Reiki has given me the tools to recognise myself, accept myself and fall in love with myself and to treat all others as I now treat myself – with respect, with love, with kindness.

But also I've come to realise that I no longer fear walking away from anything or anyone that feels negative to me. I no longer feel guilt over putting myself first and being selfish in such a way as to keep negativity away from me. I no longer look for acceptance, because I'm not afraid any more of being different or standing alone. Of course I do still get the odd doubt now and then, but I have the tools to overcome that.

Now, I'm in a place where I'm growing again, where my body is changing and I physically feel older, slightly broken, but it's OK because I still feel young at heart. I'm learning constantly about the world around me and also about me, how much I'm changing as I come to another era of my life, and I look to what future I have with a keenness I never felt before – probably because as we age, we do stop caring so much about what others think or do. I just want to live out my life with my partner in a quiet, happy space, on my terms, and I'm willing to fight for my terms.

I won't always be a professional Reiki Practitioner, but Reiki will always be my go-to resource for any cleansing or healing I require. Reiki allows me to love, to give, to be grateful, to recognise my strengths and weaknesses, and to understand myself and my place in the universe. Reiki will be to me what I need it to be, always for my highest good, to be my own unique highest potential.

How to Be Your Highest Potential with Reiki

To be able to 'be' your highest potential, you must actually find and recognise yourself at your deepest core. The cleansing and healing that Reiki brings allows you to break down all your barriers to see who you truly are – your potential, flaws and beauty, and everything that you hold within you. Reiki will always be about healing the self, first and foremost, and you must break down barriers to put yourself first.

Learning to truly recognise who you were, who you are now and who you will be is a gift that must be seen as a journey. You are on a journey of self-discovery from the moment you are born and you never stop discovering unless you stop evolving. When we let negativity, trauma, dis-ease, lack of self-discipline and lack of mindfulness take over our thoughts and feelings, we stop evolving and remain in a dark place where it's easier to hide from ourselves and remain a victim as such.

Just the smallest acknowledgement of who we are and what we have been through can help us break patterns that hold us back. It can be scary to acknowledge pain, but unless we learn from it, we allow it to control who we are and what we do.

When we connect to our deepest core, we recognise how we are all connected to each other and to the whole universe and yet we and our paths are unique. We remember that our learning will take a lifetime and that what we want and who we are today is not guaranteed to be the same tomorrow. We learn to accept ourselves and love ourselves for who we are now, and that is a gift.

It's not easy, but at the same time, it's not actually that hard. The only demons we are going to face are our own, and if we can learn to face our demons we can learn from them, from our personal experiences, to truly love, like, care for and respect ourselves.

What we need to work out is who we are and who we want to be. What do we want to do with our lives and will that really fulfil us, make us healthy and care for our well-being? When we start putting our well-being first, we are better able to deal with trauma and we are better placed to assist others in their own healing.

If you don't know or recognise yourself or your highest potential, try this little meditation to connect to your higher self, your soul.

Find yourself a quiet spot and relax into a meditation. Give yourself Reiki and imagine yourself in a bubble of cosmic love where you are completely safe and free to be yourself. Be there for yourself and breathe in love and breathe out love, letting love surround you and embrace you. Focus on your breathing and being in a bubble of love.

Now reach out to your higher self. See them appear before you in your bubble and allow their love to embrace you. Look at them and really see them. Look into their eyes and see their peace, their grace, their acceptance of what has come before and will come again. Know that you are a cosmic spirit travelling through space and time and that this life is only one of many lives. Your soul is timeless. Commune with your higher self or sit in silence, whatever feels right at that moment in time.

Then recognise that your higher self, your deepest self, is you at your highest potential.

Use all the tools in this book to find a connection to yourself and know that you have the option to go out and find other paths. The universe is vast and has so much to offer, and it is your choice where to explore and what you want to learn. Follow your instincts and trust yourself, and if you feel that you have followed a path not suited to you (I hate using the term 'wrong path'), take all the lessons you have learned and be grateful for them. Know that you can change your path and your life at your will. You have free will and you can break down barriers and you can be passionate about your path. It is yours. It is your life.

You alone are responsible for finding your highest potential, and only you can hold yourself back.

Reiki, the universal healing energy, is science, it is magic, and it is cosmic love on a very grand scale. Embrace it fully, embrace yourself fully and find your unique highest potential.

Lineage

I took all of my Reiki Degrees with Tiffany Crosara, who taught me Original Usui Reiki with both Eastern and Western philosophies. She, however, took her courses with different teachers, so I've included the lineage from her Shinpeden and Shihan Master Degree with Pamela Dini.

Original Usui Reiki

Western lineage
Mikao Usui
Dr Chujiro Hayashi
Hawayo Takata
Phyllis Lei Furumoto
Florence O'Neal
Jerry Farley
June Woods
Simon Treselyan
Marcus Hayward
Diane Whittle
Taggart King
Pamela Dini
Tiffany Crosara

Japanese lineage
Mikao Usui
Suzuki San
Chris Marsh
Taggart King
Pamela Dini
Tiffany Crosara

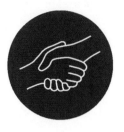

AYNI BOOKS

ALTERNATIVE HEALTH & HEALING

"Ayni" is a Quechua word meaning "reciprocity" - sharing, giving
and receiving - whatever you give out comes back to you. To
be in Ayni is to be in balance, harmony and right relationship
with oneself and nature, of which we are all an intrinsic part.
Complementary and Alternative approaches to health and well-
being essentially follow a holistic model, within which one is given
support and encouragement to move towards a state of balance,
true health and wholeness, ultimately leading to the awareness of
one's unique place in the Universal jigsaw of life - Ayni, in fact.
If you have enjoyed this book, why not tell other readers by
posting a review on your preferred book site.

Recent bestsellers from AYNI Books are:

Reclaiming Yourself from Binge Eating
A Step-By-Step Guide to Healing
Leora Fulvio, MFT
Win the war against binge eating, wake up each morning at peace
with your body, unafraid of food and overeating.
Paperback: 978-1-78099-680-6 ebook: 978-1-78099-681-3

The Reiki Sourcebook (revised ed.)
Frans Stiene, Bronwen Stiene
A popular, comprehensive and updated manual for the Reiki novice, teacher and general reader.
Paperback: 978-1-84694-181-8 ebook: 978-1-84694-648-6

The Chakras Made Easy
Hilary H. Carter
From the successful Made Easy series, Chakras Made Easy is a practical guide to healing the seven chakras.
Paperback: 978-1-78099-515-1 ebook: 978-1-78099-516-8

The Inner Heart of Reiki
Rediscovering Your True Self
Frans Stiene
A unique journey into the inner heart of the system of Reiki, to help practitioners and teachers rediscover their True Selves.
Paperback: 978-1-78535-055-9 ebook: 978-1-78535-056-6

Middle Age Beauty
Soulful Secrets from a Former Face Model Living Botox Free in her Forties
Machel Shull
Find out how to look fabulous during middle age without plastic surgery by learning inside secrets from a former model.
Paperback: 978-1-78099-574-8 ebook: 978-1-78099-575-5

The Optimized Woman
Using Your Menstrual Cycle to Achieve Success and Fulfillment
Miranda Gray
If you want to get ahead, get a cycle! For women who want to create life-success in a female way.
Paperback: 978-1-84694-198-6

The Patient in Room Nine Says He's God
Louis Profeta
A roller coaster ride of joy, controversy, triumph and tragedy;
often all on the same page.
Paperback: 978-1-84694-354-6 ebook: 978-1-78099-736-0

Re-humanizing Medicine
A Holistic Framework for Transforming Your Self, Your Practice,
and the Culture of Medicine
David Raymond Kopacz
Re-humanizing medical practice for doctors, clinicians, clients, and
systems.
Paperback: 978-1-78279-075-4 ebook: 978-1-78279-074-7

**You Can Beat Lung Cancer Using Alternative/Integrative
Interventions**
Carl O. Helvie R.N., Dr.P.H.
Significantly increase your chances of long-term lung cancer
survival by using holistic alternative and integrative interventions
by physicians or health practitioners.
Paperback: 978-1-78099-283-9 ebook: 978-1-78099-284-6

Readers of ebooks can buy or view any of these bestsellers by
clicking on the live link in the title. Most titles are published in
paperback and as an ebook. Paperbacks are available in traditional
bookshops. Both print and ebook formats are available online.

Find more titles and sign up to our readers' newsletter at http://
www.johnhuntpublishing.com/mind-body-spirit
Follow us on Facebook at https://www.facebook.com/OBooks and
Twitter at https://twitter.com/obooks